The Last Dance

Facing Alzheimer's with Love & Laughter

BY

ANN McLANE KUSTER

WITH

SUSAN McLANE

Peter E. Randall Publisher LLC
Portsmouth, New Hampshire 03802
2004

To order copies of The Last Dance
please visit www.thelastdance.org

Cover photos:
Front cover color photo by Ann McLane Kuster
Sepia photo of Malcolm, Susan, and Robin McLane taken in Norway,
1949, by David J. Bradley
Back cover and flap photos by Ken Williams, Concord Monitor

Book Design: Grace Peirce

Peter E. Randall Publisher LLC
P.O. Box 4726
Portsmouth, NH 03802
www.perpublisher.com

*Out beyond
all the wrongdoing and rightdoing,
there is a field.*

I'll meet you there.

All Things Considered
National Public Radio
Fall 2001

For my mother, Susie,
for showing us the way home

and

for my father, Malcolm,
for learning to walk on water

Praise for The Last Dance

"This is a heartfelt story about an extraordinary woman. Susan was an inspiration to me and to so many other women who jumped into the fray in the early days. She urged me to run for office and cheered my victories. Her life and this loving memoir proves that some women can have it all--a close family and a vital political life."

Madeleine Kunin
former Vermont Governor

The Last Dance is a loving tribute by a daughter to her aging mother. It is an example of how the life of the elderly can be eased by their caring children. Reading brought tears to my eyes more than once, but the writing is a help to me in facing the uncertain future. I will be much better prepared to take care of my wife should she be afflicted, or she, care of me! Sometimes I think that while we don't have "All-zheimer's," we seem to have "Half-zheimer's!"

Lowell Thomas, Jr.
Anchorage, Alaska

Susan McLane has devoted her life to improving the lives of others. For 25 years as a state legislator, Susan dedicated her career to helping women achieve their rights and freedom. In The Last Dance, Susan directs her formidable energy and passion to the greatest personal challenge of her life with the same grace and dignity that she has demonstrated her whole life. The Last Dance is a testament to Susan's optimism and commitment to others, providing hope to families who are coping with aging and Alzheimer's disease, and inspiration to women interested in making the world a better place by becoming involved in politics.

Kate Michelman, Past President
NARAL
Washington, D.C.

The Last Dance brought tears to my eyes, more of joy than of sadness because I cannot remember anyone of more good will, love and quiet guts than Susan and Malcolm McLane. The book brought back memories of their

hearty good cheer and love of all good causes. Helping get David Souter to
the U.S. Supreme Court may be Susan's greatest political achievement.

> Congressman Pete McCloskey, Jr.
> Presidential Candidate (1972)
> Palo Alto, California

We read with joy and sadness your wonderful memoir. The Last Dance *is a*
splendid book, well written and insightful into the remarkable life of a
woman who has brought so much good to so many over the years. The book
captures the essential Susan in so many ways, in particular her compassion
and capability in pursuing causes in which she believed. The Last Dance *is*
a good (but difficult) book for all of us and will be passed on to our family to
read as well.

> Dick Thornburgh
> Former Governor of Pennsylvania and
> United States Attorney General
> Washington, D.C.

This beautiful little book transcends modern medicine and technology by
tenderly sharing the relationship between a mother and her daughter. The
exquisite description of the erosion of an aging mind is poignantly sur-
rounded by a daughter's profound telling of her own efforts to understand,
comfort, and above all, love her mother. These pages will touch the heart of
anyone who has shared the travails, the humor, frustration, and fear as the
parent we once knew, slowly, before our eyes, recedes into another world.

> James W. Squires, M.D.
> President
> Endowment for Health
> Concord, New Hampshire

Ann McLane Kuster's loving tribute to her remarkable mother, Susan
McLane is a very special tale of a great woman's personal growth and
pioneering achievement on behalf of all women everywhere. Susan and
Malcolm McLane are in the first rank of progressive leaders in New
Hampshire history. Ann's book sheds special light on that journey and
constitutes an engrossing and inspiring story of Susan's courageous and
indomitable spirit.

> Walter Peterson
> Former Governor of New Hampshire

As a physician who has long specialized in the care of persons with Alzheimer's disease, I have traveled with many, many people on their journey to the "long goodbye." It is always very painful to observe an individual gradually fade under the terrible veil of confusion and chaos. At times, however, I am lucky enough to share this journey with a family so loving and strong that even Alzheimer's cannot shake its foundation, its traditions, or its grace. Such is the case with the McLanes. Susan is a remarkable woman, with a remarkable family. This wonderful book helps us see not only all that is lost in this disease but, even more, how much remains. Susan's indomitable spirit, intelligence, and charm are at the center of this story, much more than her Alzheimer's. This is how it should be, of course, but those of us who care for people with Alzheimer's disease need to remember to look beyond the illness and its symptoms, to see the person who is afflicted.

The Last Dance is also a powerful reminder that caring for someone with Alzheimer's disease may be difficult and stressful, but can be a deeply gratifying experience, as well. Ann's loving devotion to her mother is a wonderful inspiration. It will undoubtedly help others in her position see – perhaps through tears – the opportunities to remain connected to a loved one, even as the relationship changes in fundamental ways.

I would highly recommend The Last Dance to anyone who is caring for a family member with Alzheimer's. It should also be required reading for health care professionals who work with people with the disease, or their families. I have read a great many personal accounts of Alzheimer's, and this is one of the very best.

Robert B. Santulli, M.D.,
Dartmouth-Hitchcock Medical Center
Chair, Medical Advisory Council,
Alzheimer's Association of Vermont
and New Hampshire

"Through her exemplary life in politics and public service, Susan McLane has taught us so much. She stood firmly for her convictions and called things the way she saw them. In The Last Dance, her grace and courage teach us new lessons as she and her family face the challenge of Alzheimer's.

Hillary Rodham Clinton, U.S. Senator

PREFACE

A tourist remarked on a visit to New Hampshire when he first saw Lake Winnipesaukee,

"Wow, that's a lot of water."

"Yep," said the local, "and that's just the top."

In any life story, there is a lot of water on top, but a lot more if you dive below the surface to where the water is deep. *The Last Dance* is our family's story about learning to swim in the deep end of the lake when the woman we all love best, our mother, Susan McLane, slips away, one day at a time, to Alzheimer's disease.

The Last Dance began as the world's longest e-mail to my siblings. *Part One* was written in the fall of 2001, edited by New Hampshire journalist John Milne and printed in a limited edition for family and friends by Capitol Copy in Concord, New Hampshire, in January 2002. This first version of the book served an important purpose for our family and close friends coming to terms with my mother's decline. For two years, my mother read her book every day, from front to back, and then she began at the beginning again.

Part Two was written in the spring of 2004 to bring my mother's story up to the present. We are grateful to Peter Randall, Deidre Randall, and Grace Peirce of Peter E. Randall Publisher LLC in Portsmouth, New Hampshire for bringing *The Last Dance* to a wider audience. My parents are pleased to share their experience in the hope of helping others to understand aging and Alzheimer's in their own lives. We hope that by sharing our life story, we can help other families come to terms with the challenges they face, learning to love one another so much that it hurts to let go.

I'll close with these words about my mother, Susan McLane:

There are those who follow where others lead,
and there are those who blaze their own trail.

We hope Susie's story will open your heart and mind to a new approach to living well by making a difference in the world and to facing aging and Alzheimer's disease, or whatever challenge you face, with grace and courage, love and laughter.

We hope you find peace in your heart. We hope you have faith in our world. Be well.

$\mathcal{A}$CKNOWLEDGEMENTS

We live in an amazing community, where every day, walking down Main Street or down the aisle in the grocery store, someone stops to talk with my parents to offer them love and support. By sharing her story openly and honestly, my mother has opened the hearts and minds of so many people. My parents appreciate every kind word, every hug, and every smile along the way.

For two years, the Concord Regional Visiting Nurse Association staff was helpful every week, coming to the house to help my mother take a shower and assist with her "activities of daily living." Our friend Ellen Sheridan and the Alzheimer's Association of Vermont and New Hampshire have been a valuable source of support and information. Family meetings with Alzheimer's patients and their caregivers at The Birches in Concord gave my parents the opportunity to share their story and to learn from the experience of other families. Now we are blessed every day by the kindness and compassion of my mother's caregivers at Havenwood in Concord.

Our entire family has learned to support one another through this chapter in our lives. I will be forever grateful to my sister Robin McLane, who came from Portsmouth every weekend during the winter and spring of 2004, to help my father and to visit my mother. Robin and I appreciate the support and compassion of our siblings, Donald McLane and his wife Lois Garland from Twisp, Washington; Debbie and Peter Carter from Norwich, Vermont; and Alan and Alice McLane from Jackson, New Hampshire for every visit, call, and e-mail message sending their love from afar. My parents and I appreciate everyone's willingness to share our family story to help others face the challenges of aging and Alzheimer's disease.

My dear friends, Beth Moore and Lucia Kittredge, provided invaluable support and insight on long walks and talks in the hot tub late into the night about growing up an identical twin and coming to terms with Alzheimer's disease in a large family. In my special community of Hopkinton, we nurture our hearts and souls by walking and talking with friends. I am indebted to Susan Saviteer, Lisa Eberhart, Anne Smith, Mary Cowan, and Ronnie Wise for the miles of understanding behind us and the many miles more to come. I am grateful, too, to my yoga teacher, Faith Minton, and to Jane McClung at Womankind Counseling Center for bringing a map and carrying a flashlight as I make my way along this rocky trail.

Thank you to my clients and colleagues at Rath, Young and Pignatelli, P.A., for their support and understanding during these past many months, especially my amazing assistant, Suzanne Wyman, who makes my life work every day.

Most of all, I want to thank my parents, Susan and Malcolm McLane for sharing their life story so openly and honestly. Whether passing a bill in the New Hampshire Legislature, raising millions of dollars for a cause you love, or facing an illness that will literally leave you speechless, you will succeed in life if you remind yourself every day to have passion about what you do, to be patient with yourself and those around you, and above all else, to persevere. Life is short, but the days are long, and you, too, can make a difference in our world.

My sons, Zach and Travis Kuster, were my first readers before I ever imagined sharing my mother's story outside our family. Each in his own way, Zach and Travis have taught me invaluable lessons about facing life's daily challenges with grace and courage, love and laughter.

Finally, and most importantly, I count my blessings every day for my husband, Brad Kuster, who let me learn to fly, knowing that he would be there when I fell from the sky. He is a brave man and for that I love him dearly.

Contents

Preface · xi
Acknowledgements · xiii
Foreword by David Broder · xix
Introduction · xxiii
Malcolm and Susan McLane Family Tree · xxv

PART ONE

ONE
Christmas Nighties · 1

TWO
Role Reversal · 6

THREE
Fridays with Susie · 12

FOUR
Stuck in the Superlative · 16

FIVE
The First Friday — The Acceptance Speech · 21

SIX
The Zen of Motherhood · 27

SEVEN
Emergency 911 · 36

EIGHT
The Second Friday — Balance of Power · 42

NINE
Chicken Soup for the Supreme Soul · 50

TEN
Disaster Relief · 54

ELEVEN
The Third Friday — Public Servant · 61

TWELVE
The Fourth Friday — 'Crown Thy Good with Sisterhood' · 69

THIRTEEN
'Try to Remember That Day in September' · 73

FOURTEEN
The Fifth Friday — Primary Care · 78

FIFTEEN
Paradise Point · 87

SIXTEEN
The Sixth Friday — Mother Nature · 96

SEVENTEEN
Heart and Soul · 117

EIGHTEEN
Wishful Thinking · 122

NINETEEN
The Seventh Friday — 'Everybody's All American' · 124

TWENTY
The Eighth Friday — 'No Place to Hide' · 134

TWENTY-ONE
Mind, Memory, and Aging · 143

TWENTY-TWO
The Ninth and Tenth Fridays – 'Tis a Gift to Be Simple' · 149

PART TWO

TWENTY-THREE
Heaven's Gate · 161

TWENTY-FOUR
'Live Free or Die' · 164

TWENTY-FIVE
The Old Man of the Mountain · 170

TWENTY-SIX
'Day Is Done' · 176

TWENTY-SEVEN
'On Earth, as It Is in Heaven' · 181

Epilogue · 188

Book Club Discussion · 193

About the Author · 196

ℱOREWORD

For almost forty years now, the home away from home for myself and other reporters covering the New Hampshire presidential primary has been presided over by Malcolm and Susan McLane. I cannot even remember how I first fell into their hospitable grasp, but I know it was in 1964, when Nelson Rockefeller, their candidate, was running against Barry Goldwater.

Over the years, we have become close friends — a distinction I share with dozens of other Washington journalists for whom New Hampshire is a favorite stop on the campaign trail, not least because of the warm welcome that always awaits at the McLanes.

At some point along the way, I began the pleasant custom of going up to the *Concord Monitor* on primary day, having late morning coffee with its publisher, editor, and as many reporters as were back from their early-morning interviews at the polls. And after the *Monitor*, I would stop by the McLanes for a bowl of Susan's great homemade soup — and conversation about what we had seen and what we might expect when the returns came in that evening. Malcolm was always judicious in his judgments; Susan, passionate in her preferences.

It also has been our custom to pick an evening during the pre-primary weeks and drive off with a few others for dinner at the Crystal Quail, the tiny, world-class restaurant hidden off in the woods north of Concord on a road that only Malcolm can reliably find.

But the greatest treat came when I found myself in New Hampshire off-season, during the summer, when the McLane clan moves up to their "cottage" on Newfound Lake — a wonderful, rustic place complete with sauna and a seemingly endless supply of spare bedrooms.

It is there, even more than in their Concord setting, that the full force of the McLanes' personalities comes into view. Malcolm, presiding at the head of the table, every bit the pater familias — almost as if he had stepped out of Clarence Day's "Life with Father." Here the great lawyer, the wise and brave man, the shrewd judge of talent, the mentor to generations of judges and elected officials and at least one member of the U.S. Supreme Court, revels in the jibes of his children and grandchildren — and takes enormous pleasure in their company.

And Susan, who has cooked the meal and picked the flowers and done a dozen other things — all the while chatting up her friends and fellow environmental activists on the phone — is somehow engaged with every one of the young people, to say nothing of the outside guests, as if she found each one of them the best of company.

It is an extraordinary atmosphere the McLanes create, and the overwhelming sense I have had, leaving their home after every visit, is the palpable, almost overwhelming sense of love that pervades their lives. There is so much joy, so much affection, so much deep respect among them, that you depart refreshed in spirit and grateful that they have allowed you to share in their lives.

I thought of all those days and nights when reading *The Last Dance*. This, too, is a love story, a simple, straightforward but painfully honest story of how a family — and especially a mother and daughter — deal with the crushing burden of Alzheimer's. They deal with it as they have dealt with every other part of their lives, by embracing it, enfolding it into their shared experience — and then overwhelming it with their love.

I know I am biased, because of the deep affection I feel for the McLanes. But I cannot imagine anyone finishing this book without a sense of gratitude for what Annie and Susan and all their family have allowed the readers to share. Like their hospitality, it warms your heart and lifts your spirit. These people really know how to give to others what they so richly enjoy themselves—love, love, and more love.

David S. Broder
The Washington Post

INTRODUCTION

It takes a village to write a book. What began as the world's longest e-mail to my siblings soon developed into a story to share with family and close friends. As time passed, my parents and I began to realize that my mother's approach to losing her memory and self to Alzheimer's disease could help others coping with aging and Alzheimer's. Our own tears and laughter could open the hearts and heal the wounds for families coming to terms with the changes in their lives.

As we began sharing our secret hopes and fears about our lives, family and friends responded to our story with open hearts. The love and the caring of our community are simply overwhelming. We feel blessed by every hug in the supermarket, every phone call from a long-lost cousin, every letter from an old friend.

My mother has led a public life, serving for twenty-five years in the New Hampshire Legislature and running for Congress in 1980. Thousands of people know her by name and recognize her face wherever she goes. For years, she felt their pain, advocating for the mentally ill, for welfare mothers, for dignity in dying. She fought to save the environment, preserving our lakes, and protecting our wildlife. She was a tireless advocate for women in politics, raising funds and recruiting candidates. She made a difference in the lives of others. She made the world a better place for us all.

Now her world is changing. Plaques and tangles in her brain blur her memory and slow her speech. Her life is slower. Everything takes time. Still she cares about others, sending a birthday card, cooking a meal, solving the tax structure of the

State of New Hampshire. She is still making a difference in the lives of others, opening her heart and our minds to aging and Alzheimer's disease, sharing her life story. She is still making the world a better place for all.

Five million Americans have Alzheimer's disease now. In ten years, the number will grow to fifteen million. In New Hampshire, twenty thousand people have Alzheimer's, touching the lives of families all across the state. Most people have someone in their lives — a spouse, a parent, a friend — who is experiencing memory loss with aging or who has been diagnosed with Alzheimer's disease. We hope our story will help you and the people you love come to terms with failing memories and false dreams for the future. We hope you will learn to celebrate the joy in every moment. We wish you peace in your heart and faith in our world.

Last fall a friend said to me, "Annie, you are not writing a book; your mother is channeling a book through you." I have done my best to tell my mother's story. Every mother has a story to tell, from the mother who gives birth to a baby and life to a new adoptive family, to the mother who grieves over the loss of a child. Take time in your life to listen. Open your heart. Tell your mother's story. Tears and laughter, joy and pain, love and lasting peace will be your reward.

Mother's Day, May 12, 2002
Hopkinton, New Hampshire

Malcolm and Susan McLane Family Tree

John R. "Judge" McLane   Lloyd K. "Pudge" Neidlinger
    m. Elisabeth Bancroft   m. Marion Walker
    /   /
John R. McLane, Jr.   /
    /   /
Charles Bancroft McLane   Mary Neidlinger Kilmarx
    /   /
Elisabeth "Lilla" McLane-Bradley   Sally Neidlinger Hudson
    /   /
Malcolm McLane m. _____Susan Neidlinger McLane
    /   /
Mary Craig McLane   /
                             /

Susan "Robin" Bancroft McLane m. Robin Read d.
    /Marion McLane Read

Donald Walker McLane m. Joni Messer d.
    /Erik Malcolm McLane
        m. Lois Garland
    /Karissa McLane
    /Abigail McLane

Deborah McLane m. Peter Carter
    /Ashley Bancroft Carter
    /Maile McLane Carter
    /Laurel Appleton Carter

Alan McLane m. Alice Nichols
    /Laura Emily Nichols McLane
    /Carrie Nichols McLane

Ann Lloyd McLane m. Brad Kuster
    /Zachary Race Kuster
    /Travis McLane Kuster

PART ONE

FALL 2001

CHAPTER ONE

CHRISTMAS NIGHTIES

WHERE WE LIVE, the world turns a different color for every season. Autumn is filled with brilliant reds mixed with bright orange and yellow. The sky peeks through with a dazzling blue. It's beautiful, and sometimes overwhelming, like life, I suppose.

This is the story of a life filled with color, brilliant, bright, dazzling, and sometimes overwhelming. My mother, Susan McLane, has lived a beautiful life, like a party, with a long, slow dance at the end. Nobody wants the party to end. Every life is a story worth telling. This is her story, the story of her last dance.

Welcome to fall in New England, filled with color. One last big splash, before the leaves fall off the trees, the frost comes and the temperature drops until spring. For all its beauty, fall is a sign of the end of life. For every time, there is a season. This is her season.

You see, my mother has Alzheimer's disease. Every day for the past year when someone on Main Street or in the State House has asked, "How's your mother?" I have tried to find the words to tell her story. "She's doing fine, but have you heard? She's having trouble with her short-term memory." Then a few months later, I would try, "Oh, thank you for asking; you know she's headed toward a diagnosis of Alzheimer's." And then finally, simply, "My mother has Alzheimer's disease."

What are the right words? Is it like cancer, "The doctors have detected Alzheimer's"? or a cold or flu, "She's had a bout with Alzheimer's"? Gradually, I began to realize that my mother needed a word to describe what was changing in her world. Alzheimer's is the word that she has chosen. Dementia is just too creepy. So her perception has slowly become our reality.

My mother has led the way, telling friends and strangers alike, "You know, I have Alzheimer's." In May 2001, at a tribute to the McLane family, honoring three generations for community service, she turned to our friend who was hosting the dinner.

"Ruth Zax," she said, "what a lovely name. I knew a Ruth Zax thirty years ago."

Ruth responded, somewhat taken aback, "You still do, Susan, you still do and she's sitting right here next to you." The past slowly became the present and the future simply drifted away.

~

Fall is finally here after a long, hot, dry summer. The kids are back in school, with homework, spelling tests, and soccer practice filling the calendar and our life. How did my mother manage all this with five children?

When we were growing up, our lives revolved around a poster-sized calendar hanging in the kitchen, with music lessons, dentists appointments, PTA meetings, and the League of Women Voters all vying for her time and attention. All summer long, I have been thinking about my mother's amazing life, from eighteen-year-old bride to candidate for Congress, all while raising a large family and serving twenty-five years in the New Hampshire Legislature.

My mother is an avid birder with a lifelong devotion to the environment. She is a born-again feminist committed to reproductive choice for all women and dedicated to the notion that "a woman's place is in the house—the State House and the White House." She is an advocate for the mentally ill, the poor, and the disadvantaged. She is a gourmet cook who entertains effortlessly and loves nothing more than good food, cheap wine, and stimulating conversation.

But now my mother's life is changing. Her world is shrinking in both time and place. Gradually, over the past eighteen months, she has wound down her commitments, slowly letting go of the endless round of boards and committees, speeches and meetings. Week by week, she has slipped into the past, letting go of the future quietly, effortlessly, peacefully.

ॐ

Susie's world began to change in December 1999, with the Christmas nighties. With a husband, five children, four in-laws, and eleven grandchildren, Christmas has always been a big production. Over the years, her gift giving has evolved from individual presents for each person to similar presents for many.

My mother's favorite tradition is the Christmas nighties. For the past fifty years, every Christmas Eve before the reading of *The Night Before Christmas*, the children would open one present. Year after year, filled with anticipation and excitement, the present was always the same, nighties for the girls and pajamas for the boys.

With eight granddaughters in five years, the nighties came to symbolize for my parents everything that was good in the world at Christmas. Susie loved the scene of the adorable little girls in their new nighties lined up on the couch as Malcolm read *The Night Before Christmas*. Pictures were taken. Memories were made. There was peace in Susie's world. The Christmas nighties made her happy.

So in August, when she saw cute cotton nighties on sale, Susie bought eight. Then in November, when she came across the traditional plaid flannel nighties, my mother bought eight again. Except this time, she did not remember. When she found both sets of nighties in the back of her closet, we wrapped them up and warned everyone to prepare the girls for lots of nighties.

The problem was that the precious little girls were now teenagers and they did not want any nighties, let alone two apiece. Susie's world had changed once again. It turned out that teenage girls sleep in boxer shorts and T-shirts, just like the boys.

My sisters discussed at length whether to confront the nightie issue with Susie. We all engaged in the perennial Christmas debate about whether a present is designed to please the person receiving it or, more likely, the person giving it.

But this time, I realized that the question simply did not matter anymore for our family. My mother did not remember, nor did she care. In her changing world, life is beautiful, and sometimes overwhelming.

In the end, my sisters and I realized that there were no Christmas presents for any of us. So we reminded the girls to be polite and appreciative to Susie when the nighties were opened, then later to give them to the three of us and our sisters-in-law. Everyone was happy. Susie was delighted that on the eve of the new millennium, the world was once again at peace, filled with Christmas nighties.

ॐ

New Year's Eve 2000 came and went, without a whimper from the Y2K bug. But our lives started to change, in subtle and sometimes mysterious ways. When we were young and our big old house in Concord was filled with the delightful chaos of children's busy lives, we were used to our mother never finishing her sentences. The phone would ring, the dog would bark, and she would trail off to another thought, leaving us standing in the kitchen wondering what she had wanted to say. In later years, when my mother was in the legislature, serving as chair of the House Ways and Means Committee and tackling the tax structure of the State of New Hampshire, she was often in another world.

But now her mind would trail off to another era, another time in her life. The present became more and more of a challenge. She could not remember names anymore, the hallmark of a good politician. She seemed to prefer the past.

Finally, in late February 2000, I sat down on the couch at our ski house in Jackson and looked my mother right in the eyes. It seems so simple now, but at the time, it took all my courage.

With tears in my eyes, I asked her, "Momma, would you like to see a doctor to talk about your memory loss?"

Her response was like that of a child: "Oh, could I? Yes, please, I would like that very much."

I wondered if she even knew that a doctor might help her. Then I realized that I didn't know either, but I also knew that we needed to find out.

CHAPTER TWO

ROLE REVERSAL

IT WAS EARLY SPRING of 2000 after my parents returned from a trip down the Amazon, when we finally went to see a neurologist. Sitting in the doctor's waiting room with my mother for the first time in thirty years, I was suddenly aware of the role reversal. In the doctor's office, she sat up on the examining table as I watched from a chair by the desk.

The doctor performed a series of neurological tests, asking my mother to touch her finger to her nose and to walk a straight line. He reviewed the results of her MRI and EEG, explaining to us that she had suffered a minor stroke, which could be the cause of her short-term memory loss.

The doctor asked my mother if she remembered meeting him before.

"Did you go to Hanover High School?" she asked expectantly, although he was clearly twenty years younger than she was.

"No," he replied, reviewing the medical record, "we met at my office three years ago."

Then I remembered that my mother had been to a neurologist for testing when she first lost her sense of taste. I felt compelled to explain her circumstance to him.

"My mother has been in politics in New Hampshire for twenty-five years," I said. "It's no exaggeration that ten thousand people know her by name. There's no way she could remember them all."

Then my mother chimed in. "Would you have recognized me in the grocery store?" she asked. From the look on his face, I could tell that she had scored.

"No," the doctor conceded, "I would not."

Before we left, the doctor recommended that my mother take an aspirin a day to lower her chance of another stroke. He assured us that she did not yet have a definitive diagnosis of Alzheimer's disease. We both walked out of his office relieved and hopeful.

The feeling lasted throughout the summer of 2000. My mother went about her life, adapting to her short-term memory loss day by day. One trick from the campaign trail served her especially well. Whenever she ran into someone whose name she could not remember, she would throw her arms around the person and plant a big kiss on his cheek. Her theory, which proved to be foolproof, was that the person would assume that she knew him so well that she did not need to call him by name. It worked every time.

As time went by, my father began to adapt as well. In the early stages, he was in a state of denial. Whenever I tried to talk with him about my mother's memory loss, he would change the subject. I realized that acknowledging her aging was painful for him. Looking into their future together required my father to face his own mortality.

My parents had celebrated their fiftieth-wedding anniversary two summers before. They had experienced their ups and downs, as in any marriage, but now their life worked well for both of them. They were happy, and no one was inclined to rock the boat.

Our family first began to notice the transition in their roles over the telephone. Throughout our lives, my mother was in charge of making the plans. In fact, I had rarely spoken with my father by phone. Slowly, we began to notice that she was confused about dates and times and places to meet. My father would come onto the phone to clarify the arrangements.

Over time, our family communication changed completely. We would chat briefly with Susie at the beginning of the call and then talk at length with Malcolm. But everyone knew not to talk long in the morning. "Katie's back," he would say, "I have to go." My father is in love with Katie Couric, on *The Today Show*, and nobody interrupts their time together.

By September 2000, my father was completely engaged with my mother's decline. He accompanied her to the next round of doctor's visits. Slowly, he became an authority on aging, reading about dementia and the various stages of Alzheimer's disease.

I remained hopeful and made plans for a birthday party to celebrate Susie's life with family and close friends. We even bought her a "mail station" so that she could begin communicating by e-mail over the Internet. The party was fun, but Susie never even tried the "machine," as she called it. Instead, Malcolm enjoyed the messages from his grandchildren and his charitable causes.

By Thanksgiving 2000, everyone in the family realized that Susie's life was changing. She produced a magnificent turkey dinner, but then sat silent through the meal, unable to follow our lively conversation. We decided to choose names to exchange Christmas presents, rather than burden her with the task another year. Susie was delighted with the concept. We realized that we should have made the change years ago.

Gathering before Christmas to exchange presents at my house in Hopkinton, the whole family was joyful and relaxed, as though we all felt relieved of her burden. As time passed, we began to appreciate everything that Susie had done in our lives.

⌇

During the winter of 2001, we resumed our weekly trek north to ski at Wildcat Mountain. My father was one of the founders of Wildcat back in 1955, along with two Olympic ski racers, Brooks Dodge and George Macomber. Our family has shared a ski house with the Macomber family ever since. In the early years, we rented an old farmhouse and filled the rooms with mattresses discarded by St. Paul's School. Then in 1966, the two families built a ski chalet in Jackson with a perfect view of Mount Washington.

By the 1990s, "Club Max" became a three-generational getaway every weekend in winter. My husband, Brad, and I, with our boys, Zach and Travis, shared the house with Gay Macomber and her family, along with my parents most weekends. The children loved the expanded family fun, with bunkrooms, Foosball tournaments, and a crowd for every meal.

My parents loved the scene at Club Max. Gay's cute girls brought them coffee in bed every morning and crawled in under the covers for a story. During the cocktail hour, the kids bundled up and headed out sledding, just to give the grown-ups five minutes of peace. While our husbands tuned skis and cut firewood, Gay and I cooked hearty dinners with Susie and talked in front of the fire with Malcolm.

During the day, my father held forth in the ski lodge at Wildcat, reading the *New York Times*, watching out for freezing children and handing out lunch money. Malcolm finally gave up skiing, after sixty years of hiking and ski racing in the White Mountains had resulted in two knee replacements. The rest of us ski every weekend. All the kids are ski racers on the Wildcat Ski Team. Skiing is in our genes.

My mother would take one or two long runs down the Polecat, skiing like a Cadillac despite two artificial hips. She insisted on going out alone. We finally stopped worrying about her. Inevitably, Susie would return with a story of skiing all morning with some interesting man she met on the chairlift. My mother never worried about talking to strangers. In fact, she loves new people. There are no strangers in Susie's world, just folks she hasn't met yet.

☞

In late February 2001, I had surgery for torn ligaments in my knee. Rather than go home to cope with my own family, I went to my parents' condo to recover. For the first time in my life, my mother was devoted to caring just for me. She brought me a steady stream of ginger ale and homemade chicken soup. She filled the ice machine for my knee every few hours, day and night. She washed my nightie every day while I took a hot bath. Through the haze of painkillers, I basked in my mother's love and attention.

When I was young, my mother's life was filled with the delightful chaos of a large family. The legend is that I was raised by my sister Debbie, who held my hand or lugged me around on her hip. Then, when my mother ran for the legislature, I had my own teenage life. We would talk about taxes and politics at the dinner table, but not about my life, my friends, my thoughts. Later in life, we were both too busy to talk about our lives. My mother was running the State Senate and I was juggling two babies of my own with my law practice.

But now our lives were on hold. Susie's world was shrinking to a simple, domestic life of cooking and laundry, while I was laid up by the surgery, loving every minute of her time and attention. In the evenings, we lay on my parents' big double bed and watched movies together, *Butch Cassidy and the Sundance Kid* and other flashbacks to an earlier era. For one brief moment in our lives, we were one, without a care in the world, bonded together. I found peace in my heart.

CHAPTER THREE

FRIDAYS WITH SUSIE

IN MAY 2001, the doctors pronounced my mother's diagnosis to be "probable Alzheimer's disease." Based on her medical history, current medical exam, and neuro-psych testing, my mother's memory loss and functional difficulties met the criteria for a diagnosis of Alzheimer's. She accepted the doctor's conclusion graciously, but the rest of our family needed time to come to terms with the news.

In late June, as we gathered for our annual "Cousins Camp" at our home on Newfound Lake, Susie became intent on photocopying all of her political speeches for her daughters and granddaughters. She presented the copies to each of us with a personal inscription, her own private inspiration as though she was passing on the torch, hoping we would carry on her many worthy causes.

In July 2001, settled in with my father in the little cottage down the lake, my mother spent her time rereading all the journals she had kept of their travels, reminiscing about their wonderful life together. Every day, my parents would go for a drive, winding aimlessly over the back roads through the White Mountains and along the lakes and streams of northern New Hampshire.

In the evenings, my mother would cook simple, delicious meals. My parents would eat together on the porch watching the glorious sunset over the lake. Fresh corn and new potatoes for dinner became corn chowder for lunch the next day. Poached salmon appeared again as salmon pâté on crackers for an hors d'oeuvre. Family and friends came to visit. Slowly we all came to terms with the next chapter of their life.

By midsummer, my parents had news to share with us. They had applied to live at Kendal, a retirement community in Hanover where Malcolm's sister Lilla and brother Charles live. The idea came to them over lunch with Lilla, and they applied the very next day.

During the interview, Malcolm diplomatically told the woman that "Susan has had a minor stroke and her memory is limited."

In her typical candor, Susie chimed right in, "I have Alzheimer's, you know."

The woman kindly replied, "So do many of our residents. We'll take care of you here."

We were all relieved. Our uncertainty and fear about the future began to slip away. My parents were delighted, as if they had just been accepted into college. There was peace and order in our world once again.

When she filled out the personal questionnaire for Kendal, my mother did not hesitate to answer the questions with complete honesty.

In response to the question "What are your plans for the future?" she wrote simply, "Nothing. My life is in the past."

When asked, "Will you miss your family and friends?" my mother wrote, "No, my family will be here and I have friends, but I can't remember their names." Her words were direct and to the point, without pain or anger or frustration.

Responding to the question "Do you have any regrets about your life?" she wrote, "No, I am relieved that I did not win when I ran for Congress."

I began to wonder how many of us will feel that way. When all is said and done, will we have regrets looking back on the choices we have made, the decisions that have framed our lives? What was it about my mother's life, or Alzheimer's disease, that gave her such peace of mind?

I wanted to tell my mother's story before her memory slipped away completely. I wanted to understand her past and to come to terms with her future, as she has so peacefully. I hoped that her candor about Alzheimer's could open up the world of aging just as the book *Tuesdays with Morrie* has for death and dying.

In August 2001, I presented the idea to my parents. Beginning in September, I would come to their house on my day off every Friday with a tape recorder and Susie could tell me the story of her life.

I watched my parents' expressions closely for their reaction. My mother smiled, with a twinkle in her eye, looking pleased with the idea. My father said simply, with tears in his eyes and hope in his heart, "We'll call it 'Fridays with Susie.'" It was then that I knew this book was meant to be.

≈

So here I am, full of anticipation, arriving at my parents' condominium in East Concord on the first Friday in September with a tape recorder, an open mind, and a light heart. Driving from my home in Hopkinton to their neighborhood, I remember every house on the block.

I am suddenly flooded with memories of my mother's 1988 State Senate campaign, the summer that my older son, Zach, was born. She was intent on having a photo of her talking with a constituent for her campaign brochure. So I lugged the baby in the car seat with the camera as we went door-to-door, looking for the perfect moment.

Finally, we found that moment when a young mother answered the door. Susie instantly became engaged in a heart-to-heart conversation about the woman's children and their education in the public schools, her husband and his job in construction, her parents and their health care in the nursing home. This woman's worries were my mother's world. As I took the picture, I suddenly saw Susie's world in a whole different light.

Driving by that house today, I wonder how that woman's world has changed over the years and who will ever tell her story. Then I realize that this story is for her, and for every woman or man whose life has been shaped by children, spouses, parents, and the everyday cares of making the world a better place for us all.

CHAPTER FOUR

Stuck in the Superlative

As I walk into the kitchen, my mother embraces me with a big hug and a warm smile. Her hair is thin and white, her skin is soft, almost translucent, and her eyes are twinkling. She's clutching a present in her hands like a child.

"This is for you, all the way from Alaska. I can't believe that I forgot your birthday. Did anyone feature you?" my mother asks.

I kiss her on the cheek and hold her face in my hands, looking into her eyes and feeling her love. Her youngest child turns forty-five years old, and after all these years, my mother is still worrying about whether anyone has featured me on my birthday.

I open the small bag and find three pairs of earrings, bright and dangling.

"Thank you, Momma, these are beautiful. Don't worry about it. You were just getting home from a long trip. Brad and the boys featured me with breakfast in bed and dinner out," I explain.

But I know from the look in her eyes that my mother is sad about forgetting my birthday. We both know that remembering birthdays is just one more thing in her life that is slipping away.

My mother is pleased and proud to show me her journal of the trip to visit my brother Donald and his family in the North Cascades and the cruise up the Inland Passage to Alaska. I am impressed by the detail and clarity of her writing and by the pictures on each page of the people and places along the way.

For years, my mother has kept meticulous journals of her travels, from the vacation trips to Europe and around the world with my father to her legislative junkets to Japan, Korea, and South Africa. I am pleasantly surprised that she can still write down the details of every day.

Over the years, the journals have recorded the places my parents saw and the people they met, and, in a particular code about food and drink, their moods day by day. "Drinks in our room and a delicious dinner on the town" signifies a good day on the trip. "Hot bath and long nap, then drinks and dinner with friends" means that the day was strenuous, but they met new people and were happy.

"Bourbon in the bath" is the cryptic key to sheer exhaustion or misery. She was raised on the expression, "If you can't say anything nice, don't say anything at all." So in Susie's world, "bourbon in the bath" is as bad as it gets.

As the Alzheimer's disease has progressed, we have coined an expression in our family: "Susie is stuck in the superlative." Every meal is the "most delicious I've ever tasted!" and every sunset is "the prettiest I've ever seen!" The irony is that she completely lost her sense of taste three years ago, but Susie's optimism and good cheer have taken on a life of their own.

Perhaps when you cannot remember what you ate for breakfast, then lunch is the best meal you have ever eaten. Perhaps Susie is just living in the moment and finding joy in the simple pleasures of life.

The journal of the trip to Alaska is a testament to my mother's optimism. The visit with Donald and his family was a great success, but the boat trip was cold and rainy, and my parents were sick most of the time. Traveling was problematic from the start, rising at the crack of dawn without an alarm clock and rushing to the Manchester airport, only to find that the plane was four hours late.

No problem for Susie. "It didn't make *any* difference!" she writes. "We took a shuttle to Boston, free because we are *First Class* on our frequent flier miles!"

My parents finally landed in Seattle six hours later than expected. Then they drove in heavy traffic through the city and in rain and dense fog over the North Cascades pass.

Susie exclaims upon arriving at the Sun Mountain Lodge at midnight, "3 a.m. *our* time! 22 hours without a real sleep! Did our room and bed feel perfect!"

My parents loved the visit with Donald; his wife, Lois; son, Erik; and daughters, Karissa and Abigail. My brother, a former teacher and logger with a philosophy degree from Brown University, now builds second homes in the North Cascades for dot-com millionaires and diplomats. The summer of 2001, before starting college, Karissa was his crew, learning the construction trade. My parents are proud of them both.

Susie writes, "Went to the house that Donald is building. Karissa was there working and doing a great job, according to Donald. It is up on a hill, all alone, with a view of *all* the mountains like I've *never* seen!"

The food code was glowing during the visit to Twisp. Susie raves, "Had the granola and cream breakfast sitting in the dining room with the view spread out before us. (Cost $29 for breakfast—extra for coffee, $2 per orange juice!) This is a fancy place!"

Later in the day she writes, "Another perfect picnic lunch with Donald and Karissa! The view this time was spectacular!"

After dinner she writes, "All 6 of us had something different—the girls' salad and hors d'oeuvres and Donald had the steak. We shared desserts. It was the perfect end to our two day visit!" All in all, everyone had a very successful family time.

The Lindblad cruise from Sitka to Juneau was more of a challenge. Susie's journal continues in the superlative by day, with sightings of whales, birds and grizzly bears, but the nights were often miserable.

On the last day Susie finally acknowledges, "A bad night. Malc coughed all night and I was sick. But the morning sun made it all better. The first sun we've seen in 10 days! Our criteria up to now has been—if it isn't pouring rain, it's pleasant!"

Reading my mother's account of the trip, I wonder how someone so positive copes with adversity at all. Perhaps with Alzheimer's disease, misery is the memory that fades first.

ॐ

In Susie's world, there are no bad words left. I remember calling her from California Christmas Eve 2000 when I tore the ligaments of my knee in a skiing accident on the final day of a family vacation on Lake Tahoe. We were gathered for dinner at my cousin's house, celebrating the holidays with shrimp scampi and plenty of good cheer. Lying on the couch with my knee on ice and in a brace, I told my mother over the telephone the story of my accident.

My son Zach and I had been skiing off-piste on steep, rocky terrain at Sugar Bowl. All week, I felt like a teenager, chasing my cousins Jim, Jake and Bill with my boys, Zach and Travis, through the trees and down the steepest trails. But by two o'clock on Christmas Eve, I turned back into a middle-aged mom. As I tried to make a sharp turn, I fell down a steep, narrow ravine. I heard the snap and knew that my knee was injured. Then I slid headfirst thirty feet toward a pile of rocks, until Zach skied across my path to stop me.

Listening to the drama, my mother was completely at a loss for words. "Oh, sweetie," she said, and then after a long pause, "that's something."

I waited for a negative adjective. She tried again.

"That's something . . . , isn't it?" was all she could say.

With no negative words left, this nightmare for me was simply "something" for my mother, nothing more, nothing less.

All winter and spring, through the surgery and long recovery, I often thought of my mother's reaction. Whenever my knee hurt or I felt bad or sad, I would think of Susie and say to myself, "That's something, isn't it?"

Mysteriously, the pain would simply slip away. I'm learning from my mother to let the memory of misery fade first.

CHAPTER FIVE

THE FIRST FRIDAY: THE ACCEPTANCE SPEECH

WHEN WE FINISH opening presents and reading the journal, I open my bag of "Show and Tell." I have four photos to share with my mother. Dartmouth College has returned two old photographs after reproducing them for the new McLane Ski Lodge dedication last winter. One picture is of Malcolm schussing across the finish line of the Dartmouth Carnival downhill in 1946. The other is of his parents, Judge, a life trustee of Dartmouth, and Elisabeth, gliding silently through a snowy forest on Mount Tremblant in the late 1930s. Skiing has been our life for four generations. My mother is happy to revisit the memories of good times gone by.

The other two photos are of Susan and Malcolm when they were young, borrowed by *Business New Hampshire* magazine for a birthday tribute. My mother's eyes light up when she sees her picture with her identical twin sister, Sally, in the September edition of the magazine under the caption, "Can you guess who this is?"

"Do you know which one is you?" I ask her.

"No, I can't tell," she replies wistfully.

When we were young, we loved to guess who was who in pictures of the twins. Now I realize that it doesn't matter anymore. Susan and Sally are one and the same at that age, identical twins, one girl holding Raggedy Ann and the other holding a little black dog. Two girls, one identity, together forever.

As I set up the tape recorder, my mother says, "I've been wandering around this house all morning just looking back to all my years."

I know she means the pictures and memories throughout the house, decades of family photos, honors and awards, piles of mail, an endless stream of her life.

"I'm just saying, 'I'm over with the whole thing,' " my mother declares.

Just like that, so succinct and complete. I know from her expression that she is talking about her life. I know that the time has come to tell her story.

My mother settles into her chair by the fireplace. With tears in my eyes, I say, "I would like you to tell your story and then we can write about it. You can pick wherever you want to start."

My mother looks at the tape recorder, then she looks at me. She begins.

My twin sister was the most valuable part of my life. We were together all the time. We didn't fight for years and years.

When we were thirteen years old, we got our period for the first time. I got it first in the bathroom upstairs. Then Sally called from the third floor and she had gotten it, too. Mother explained it all to me and then went downstairs. She called the doctor while Sally was sitting on the john because she was so surprised. The doctor said "that's the sign of identical twins!"

My mother brings me an old photo of her first-grade class and points to twin girls in the front row. "Here we are. The two of us, always together," she says proudly.

"Can you tell which one is you?" I ask.

"No," she responds. "I don't know."

"Look at the ringlets in your hair," I say. "Who did your hair in the morning? Your mother or the maid?" I ask.

"My mother," she says fondly.

"Who else do you know in the picture?" I ask.

"I know everybody," my mother says confidently.

"Who do you recognize?" I wonder aloud.

"Here is . . . (pause) . . . Bowler," she says haltingly.

"Patsy Bowler?" I ask, remembering the name from my own childhood.

"Yes, Patsy Bowler. That's Andy . . . (pause) . . . I can't remember any of their names now. But I recognize every face. I can tell you exactly where they all lived in town."

My mother continues talking about her early years growing up in Hanover.

> *We grew up in Hanover where my father was the Dean of Dartmouth College. We went to the SAE house every day. We became excellent at pool! . . .* [she pauses, searching for the words to describe her childhood] *. . . I have some pictures of what we did when we were young.*
>
> *We were ski racers. Andrea Mead won three gold medals. She was a very good friend of ours. Sally was on the Olympic team, too. But I was having my third baby, so I was never in the Olympics.*
>
> *One of the best things that ever happened to me was to be with Sally before she died. I was retired from the legislature*

and Malcolm and I went around the world. I would have been so horrified if Sally had died when I was around the world. When I got to California, she was dying of cancer. I never came home because she wanted me to stay with her. I wasn't in the legislature and I didn't have anything else to do, so I stayed with her.

I couldn't do anything about her dying, except to be there with her. I have discovered that half of the grief about death is guilt. I didn't have any guilt when Sally died. I stayed with her for two and a half months. When she died, I wasn't sad.

I remember it all, starting with the phone call in mid-December 1994 with my mother in Hawaii. She was so excited to be coming home for Christmas after four months traveling around the world.

"Mom, when you get to Sally's, you won't want to come home," I said, knowing by then how sick Sally was.

My mother was undeterred. "But she was skiing at Thanksgiving. I'm sure she'll be fine. We'll be home in a few days. Then I can come back out to California in January after the holidays."

But when my parents arrived in Sacramento, Sally did not want Susan to leave. So my mother stayed, sending Malcolm home on his own. Living with Sally through the endless rounds of doctor's visits and chemotherapy treatments, my mother watched her identical twin sister decline day by day. Cooking her simple yet delicious meals, washing her sheets and nighties, bathing her and holding her in the night, Susie came to terms with letting go of her twin sister and losing a part of herself.

My mother came home for a week at Christmas. I remember how happy she was that Sally played golf on Christmas Day with her family. I went out to spend New Year's with my aunt, to give my mother a break and to say my own good-byes. Sally and I talked and laughed while she told me stories and family secrets.

One night, I woke up to my aunt moaning, so I took her to the hospital. Sally regaled the emergency room staff with stories about her Olympic past. But when the doctor showed me the MRI, I knew that the cancer had spread throughout her body. As he handed me the morphine, the doctor said, "Take her home and use this to keep her comfortable. It's so sad when this happens to such a wonderful person."

When we got home, I made cheese omelets and served mimosas to Sally wearing her new red cashmere sweater. I held my cousin Jake as he wept in my arms in the kitchen. Then we all settled in on the couch and planned Sally's memorial service. My aunt told us who would speak and what music to play. I had visions of Sally sitting in the middle of a large circle of family and friends, wearing her red cashmere sweater and soaking in the accolades about her amazing life.

My aunt Sally was an Olympic skier who raised three sons on her own in Squaw Valley, teaching skiing and selling real estate to make a living. When her boys were grown, Sally moved to Sacramento to follow the family passion, politics. She worked in the California State Senate and became an environmental activist. Her sons were all ski racers, too. The youngest, Bill, raced on the U.S. Ski Team in the 1988 Calgary Olympics.

Sally was loved and respected by family, friends, and colleagues. Over brunch that day, we talked about her will. My aunt made a list of who would receive all her worldly possessions. Her time had come. Her life was in order.

My mother arrived the day I left and stayed until the very end. Sally finally died on Valentine's Day at home in her own bed, with Susie and Bill holding her in their arms. They cried together, and as Sally took her last breath, Bill said, "Let go, Mom, let go. You're at the top of a long snowfield. Just let 'em run."

◡

Later on, as I am winding up our first Friday taping, I ask my mother, "How do you feel about losing your memory?"

Well, I feel that my life is over. I do feel good about the life that I have led. But I really feel that life is over now.

I am reminded of my mother's own words, "half of the grief about death is guilt." Susie has no guilt. She has led a good life, a productive life, and a meaningful life. Now she is ready to let go of it all, to pass the torch.

My mother accepted the death of her identical twin sister, Sally. Now she is accepting that her own life is coming to an end. I am beginning to accept her philosophy. I can't do anything about my mother aging, except to be here with her. It feels right for me. I hope it helps her, too.

CHAPTER SIX

THE ZEN OF MOTHERHOOD

DURING THE WEEK, I am an adoption lawyer and a lobbyist in the New Hampshire Legislature, but on the weekends I am a soccer mom. My sons, Zach and Travis, have games scheduled every Saturday and Sunday this fall. Rather than getting stressed out, I am working on the "Zen of the Soccer Mom," following my mother's example of living in the present and appreciating what life has to offer.

With coffee in hand, I join the baby-boomer crowd on the sidelines, joking with the dads and bonding with the moms. Brad and I cheer as Zach makes another save in goal and Travis scores on a perfect pass in front of the net. We are blessed. We both feel grateful simply to enjoy the moment.

On Sunday, while Brad takes the boys to another game, I drive up to Newfound Lake to meet my parents for lunch and a swim. The day is unseasonably hot. The swim in the cool, clear lake feels refreshing. We talk about plans for the lake house next summer, scheduling the cousins and paying the bills.

Over lunch, we discuss the perennial topic in our family, the tax structure of the State of New Hampshire. In one moment, my mother confuses the words for asparagus and celery for the tuna fish. In the next, she talks about oil and taxes in Alaska and how our neighboring states have both an income tax and a sales tax. Her lifelong effort to pass an income tax in New Hampshire is one topic that holds my mother's attention. But often she just sits in silence, listening to our conversation.

After our swim, we talk about the tennis match at the U.S. Open between the Williams sisters, Venus and Serena. I ask my mother, "How did you feel when you were ski racing against Sally?"

"I preferred for her to win," she replies. "I had a boyfriend and she didn't," she says proudly, pointing at Malcolm.

"But the last time Sally and I raced, at the Schneider Cup at Cranmore when we were in our sixties, I won. Sally said it was because I weighed twenty pounds more than she did, but she smoked and I didn't. I skied faster and I won!" Susie looks proud and pleased with the memory.

Malcolm was the captain of the Dartmouth Ski Team. When I was a freshman at Mount Holyoke, I won the Women's Eastern Ski Championships. I was president of my freshman class.

Then in the spring I became pregnant, so I married Malcolm. He was a Rhodes scholar. He said he didn't want to go to England for two years without me. He had been a prisoner of war. He didn't want to be alone ever again. . . . And so, . . . there it was.

I wouldn't have wanted to go four years to college. I really felt grateful to move to England with Malcolm. So I became a mother, for years and years and years. I grew up at Dartmouth, where there was a difference in how you were treated if you were a woman. Then I had five babies. He didn't use any birth control or anything, so I had five babies. I just did them and that was it.

Robin was my oldest. I have not ever said this. Do you think Robin knows that I was pregnant? [Susie asks me, looking concerned. "I think she does now, but not when she was growing up," I reassure my mother. She seems relieved.] *I'll never forget. I had ridden my bicycle all fall right up to the last day, so I had the baby in an hour and a half. Then they put me to bed for ten days. I could hardly walk at the end!*

The first day, they brought me the baby in the morning. I just looked at her and thought "this is so real." Then they said, "you are going to nurse her." I said, "I don't know anything about nursing." And they said, "She's your baby, not ours!" I've never forgotten that. I nursed all of my babies.

I nursed Alan right up to when he was nine months old. I had been in bed with two broken legs from a ski accident the year before. When I got pregnant again, the doctor offered me an abortion but I said no. I was pregnant on crutches right up to the time Alan was born. I stayed in bed every morning and nursed him for hours [she is smiling]. *Malcolm got up and fed the other children and got them off to school.*

I am amazed by my mother's life and by her candor in telling the story. I can't even imagine being a mother at age nineteen or having four babies in six years, let alone two broken legs at the same time and then being pregnant on crutches. Now I understand why my mother stayed in bed nursing her babies as long as possible. At least then she could have five minutes of peace.

"What did you think about mothering?" I ask. I open this subject with some trepidation, but I know I need to understand my mother in order to understand my own mothering.

I remember completely when you kids were growing up. [She goes to the mantel and points to the pictures of our family growing up in the 1950s and '60s.] *There they all are, five children. There you are, right there, the youngest.*

I just felt that the children were it. I remember that I was completely involved with them. I remember the Christmas cards from all these pictures. I knit all of the sweaters that you were all wearing.

"How did you do all that?" I ask in amazement.

I stayed home all day. All I did was cook and care for the children. I walked down to Souther's Market every day because we only had one car until we had all five children. I walked down and back with two of the children in the stroller to buy the dinner every day.

I never went to a supermarket. We didn't have a supermarket in those days, until the A&P opened down by the State House. Then when I got a car, I went down to the A&P every day to get the dinner. I would go over to watch the legislature from the balcony.

"Why?" I ask. "What was the draw?"

It was politics and it was interesting to Malcolm. That was the beginning of it.

I thought I was having my sixth baby. They asked me to be president of the League of Women Voters. I said I would wait a week to decide. At the end of the week, I discovered that I was not pregnant. So I got on to the new life.

Malcolm didn't realize until I got to the legislature that I was as smart as he was and that I was into politics. That is what

*is so different about my having Alzheimer's. He is completely
kind to me.*

*I think he married me because I was eighteen and he was
in charge. He was the Rhodes scholar and he knew everything.
All through the time that I was having five babies, he was in
charge. He was in charge of the money. He was in charge of
moving to the new house. He was in charge of everything. And
I just went along with it.*

"Did you ever regret that or resent him?" I wonder.

*No, I didn't back then. Then when I got to the legislature,
I just thought, "I know more about this than he does." I was
different in those days. Now I'm back to where I was before.*

"Did he get involved in parenting?" I ask, curious about my
parents' roles in raising the children.

*I was in charge in the house. He was completely helpful.
When he came home, it was just the kids, and that's what it
was. He would put the kids to bed while I washed the dishes.
I never once thought that I couldn't manage five kids. I never
felt that I had any negative feelings about the five kids. I
thought it was fun and I thought it was my job.*

I am overwhelmed by the notion of raising five children, yet
intrigued by her response. "What did you enjoy most about
having five kids?" I ask. My mother thinks for a moment, then
she answers:

*I skied and taught skiing. That was fun! I organized ski les-
sons in White Park for all the children in the neighborhood.*

I remember the scene like it was yesterday. Dozens of children bundled in sweaters, parkas, and knit hats, learning to ski
right in the middle of town in White Park. When we were in ele-
mentary school, my brother Alan and I would wear our itchy

ski pants and old lace ski boots to Dewey School, then walk across the street after school to teach ski lessons in the park.

"Bend zee knees, two dollars please!" was my mother's refrain, as we taught the children how to schuss down the slopes on wooden skis with bear-trap bindings. They loved the story of my brother Donald when he was a little boy just learning to ski. My mother would tell him to keep his legs parallel, but he was confused. "Mom, is that the cookie that grown-ups eat when they drink beer?" No wonder Donald was struggling, trying to make his legs look like a pretzel on skis.

ༀ

I remember the fun times, too, but I wonder about my mother's perception of the stage in our lives when I was twelve and she was first elected to the House.

"How did your parenting change when you first went off to the legislature?" I ask cautiously.

> *You were all grown up. You were the one who told me that. I'll never forget it as long as I live. I was waiting for you on the porch when you came home from school on the first day of seventh grade. You said to me, "Mother, get a life!"*
>
> *I never thought about you after that. Robin was in college at that time. Donald was away at school. The rest of you were just grown.*
>
> *I cooked supper every night. When I was in the legislature, Malcolm said he was glad that we lived in Concord, so that I would be home for supper every night. The gals in the legislature from Hanover stayed down in a motel during the week and left their families at home.*

"How did you juggle it all? How did you stay involved in your kids' lives while you were in the legislature?" My mother

32

looks puzzled, as though this question has never crossed her mind. She answers slowly, contemplating her response.

> *I think that the independence from me was a good thing.* [She pauses.] *If I had been home cooking and such, it would have been a whole different thing.* [She pauses again.]
> *"Mother, get a life."* . . . *That was it.* [She is smiling now, looking at me.]

Having heard this story my whole life, I often wonder whether I did say such a thing. I may have, or at least my mother may have heard the words she wanted to hear. I do remember once talking with my sister-in-law Joni, who left college her freshman year to marry my brother Donald, the day after Christmas of his senior year in high school.

Donald and Joni's son, Erik, was born five months later in May 1969. I became an aunt at age twelve and my mother became a grandmother at age thirty-nine. When my mother objected to being called Grandma, Erik gave her the name Susie, which she has been called fondly by our family ever since. I was so excited when Donald and Joni moved with Erik into our house in Concord for the summer. In the fall, they went off to Providence, where Donald began his freshman year at Brown.

I recall talking with Joni about my mother's new life in the legislature and how she was never home after school.

"Annie, you're lucky," Joni said. "Your mother has a life. That's much better than the girls whose mothers are waiting when they get home to hear about their day in school."

I especially remember the feeling I had when I realized that Joni knew all about counting her blessings. Her mother had died of cancer when she was in seventh grade.

అ

As I listen to my mother's memories of her life, I wonder what advice she would have for her eight granddaughters.

"What would you tell the girls about trying to balance it all?" I ask her, hoping her insight will give me perspective on my own life.

My mother thinks for a long time before responding. Her answer is succinct and to the point:

Finish college before you get married.

"Would you tell them to have so many children?" As the youngest of five children, this question has always been on my mind.

No. I would have one or two. Robin had one and everyone else had two. Debbie had three, but it was because she was married to a nice guy who would help.

"What would you tell them about working or staying home when the kids were little?" I ask. She thinks for a minute before answering.

I would say that they should decide that. [She pauses to think.] You were a lawyer already, so you went off because that was your law practice. Debbie taught school for a long time. Then she stayed home after she had her babies. She had three and that was much different than two. Robin ran for the legislature when her daughter was born. Then she went back to work later. [She pauses.] But I think it is all their decision, not mine.

My mother's response is just right. I am struck by her humility. With so many more options open to women in the world now, the choices in our lives are daunting. Each one of us must make the decisions that will frame her own life. My mother is satisfied with her choices. Now she is content to let us make our choices, to let us dance to our own tune.

"I think you have good advice, Momma," I say softly, as I give her a big hug. "I think it's nice for you to share it."

CHAPTER SEVEN

EMERGENCY 911

IT'S A VERY NORMAL Tuesday morning. I empty the dishwasher, drink my coffee, and talk with the boys over breakfast about packing the backpacks with lunches and homework and getting to soccer practice this afternoon. The sky is bright blue, the air is clear. September has taken hold of our lives once again. As I drive to work, I count my blessings, grateful to be living in the moment.

Coming up the stairs in the law firm, I greet our receptionist, Cindy, whose contagious good cheer can make anyone's day better. But Cindy's face is filled with horror.

"Annie, have you heard? A plane has crashed into the World Trade Center! They think it might be terrorists," Cindy says with great alarm.

As I round the corner to my office, my assistant, Suzanne, looks equally stricken.

"We were watching on the TV upstairs when another plane hit the other tower and exploded like a bomb," Suzanne says, fear in her eyes.

My heart races as I frantically search my mind to account for everyone in our family and our close friends.

All morning long the news filters into our lives. News flashes and rumors make the rounds in the office. A plane has crashed into the Pentagon. The White House has been evacuated.

As the world around us copes with the chaos, Suzanne and I go about making the arrangements for a private adoption. The call comes in that the birth mother has signed her consent to adoption in court. The adoptive parents can pick up the baby this afternoon.

Late in the morning, as the horror begins to sink in, I call my mother. Susie is distracted on the telephone.

"The Kirby guy is here showing me how it works. I'm going to give it to you for Christmas," she says.

I have no idea what she is talking about, but I realize that the terrorist attack has not yet entered Susie's world.

"I love you, Mom. I'll call back later," is all I say.

My client and I are dazed and distracted at lunch. The news is on the radio in the deli. Strangers talk freely about their fears. Our strategy for the afternoon legislative hearing seems trivial and beside the point. We talk about our children and how we will ever feel safe again.

"When I was thirteen, I read the book *The Andromeda Strain,*" I recall, reliving the nightmare end-of-the-world scenario of my teen years.

"For years, with all the Cold War fears and the threat of nuclear war, I thought that the world would not be safe enough for me ever to have children. Now, here I am with two sons, ages thirteen and ten."

"I just don't want my children to be in a war," my client responds, thinking about his four young boys. The thought of my boys going to war has never even crossed my mind.

Everyone is talking about the events of the day and trying to come to terms with the trauma. A TV cameraman is setting up his equipment on the State House lawn. We talk about the drama unfolding in New York and Washington. Another plane has crashed in western Pennsylvania, perhaps en route to an attack on the White House or the U.S. Capitol. The cameraman looks me right in the eye and says, "The world will never be the same again."

I call my mother again. Now she knows about the terrible news. "I'm going home to meet the boys after school. Why don't you come over for dinner?" I ask, just wanting my world to feel safe.

Brad and I talk on the phone about whether the boys should watch the news on TV and what is the best way to help them cope. This day will change all of our lives in some unforeseen way. I keep thinking back to the Kennedy assassination and the *Challenger* launch, where I was and what I was thinking about the world and about life and death and disaster.

Then I think about my mother's life and how she experienced tragedy. I remember as a little girl when my mother took us to greet President Kennedy at the airport in Concord. Years later, when she served in the Senate, my mother was a frequent guest in Christa McAuliffe's class on women in government at Concord High School. After Christa died in the *Challenger* disaster, my mother sponsored legislation to create the Christa McAuliffe Planetarium to honor the teacher's courage and commitment to education. I wonder if my mother is having these same thoughts today.

I pick up the boys at the school bus stop. We talk about why the attack happened, how this could happen, and what will happen next. We talk about the flight paths of the planes and how the cross-country flights were filled with fuel. Passenger airplanes became missiles and powerful bombs. The innocence of our lives fades quickly. We feel vulnerable in a new way.

Zach and Travis think up solutions to make us all feel safe. "I know, Mom, how about armed soldiers on every flight to protect the pilots and passengers?" they ask. This morning the idea would have seemed un-American, but now it makes perfect sense.

We talk about living in New Hampshire and being safe here. Then we call our friends in New York and Connecticut to make sure that everyone is okay. Laura Delano, an actress and massage therapist in Manhattan, reports that all her family are home safely. Our friend Jim made it home to New Canaan on the train, but his wife, Wendy, is an EMT headed into the city with her ambulance crew.

"We love you," I say with tears in my eyes, wishing that all will be well again soon.

Then Susie arrives in my kitchen with her arms full of food. My mother never arrives anywhere empty-handed. From her bag she pulls out an entire dinner—potatoes, peas, and some mystery meat.

"It's lamb from last night. It will be delicious warmed up again," she says with confidence. But I'm not entirely convinced, so I make a shrimp stir-fry, too.

We sit on the deck in the late afternoon sun, soaking in the view of the mountains and feeling the peace surround us. The shock is slowly sinking into our hearts and minds, but for now we feel only numbness.

When I ask my mother about her day, she talks about watching the horrific images on television of the World Trade Towers burning and then collapsing.

"Unbelievable. Simply unbelievable," is all she can say.

Our family and friends are safe, but we grieve for the victims and their families. We grieve for our loss of innocence.

When I ask my mother how she is feeling about her life, she says, "Malcolm is being so kind to me now that I can't remember a thing." Then she adds with a wink, "He always did think I was dumber than he was!"

Susie continues, "But we had our first fight today. I want to buy it, but it cost thirteen hundred dollars and he doesn't think I need it . . ." Her voice trails off. My mother cannot remember the word for "it." She tries again, but without success.

"Oh, well, if I can't even remember the word, perhaps I don't need to buy it!" she says, laughing.

"What does it do?" I ask, trying to be helpful.

"Cleans the rugs," she replies, demonstrating with her hands.

"A vacuum cleaner?" I suggest. "How could a vacuum cleaner cost thirteen hundred dollars?" I ask incredulously.

"Why? Do you think that's a lot?" Susie says innocently. "I want to buy it for you for Christmas, and then I will leave it to my daughters."

I don't even vacuum, I'm thinking, and who would leave a vacuum cleaner in her will? I can't imagine, but then, this is Susie's world. Maybe my mother wants to make my life easier or maybe she wants to leave behind something that is hers. I know my mother cares and wants to help. But I can only imagine my father's reaction to a thirteen-hundred-dollar vacuum cleaner.

ᣔ

That night, as I tuck Travis into bed, I rub his back and tell him that we are safe, here in New Hampshire.

"What will happen next?" he wonders aloud.

I try to sound reassuring when I say, "Well, if we can find the people who are responsible for the attack, we will retaliate."

"But Momma, retaliation isn't a good thing, is it?" he asks in a small voice in the dark.

"Not this morning it wasn't," I say, "but now I just don't know. It's hard to say what's right or wrong anymore."

CHAPTER EIGHT

The Second Friday: Balance of Power

W E WAKE UP Wednesday morning to the reality of our lives. The news is grim. All the passengers on the four hijacked flights perished. Many more people died when the World Trade Towers collapsed, including several hundred police and firefighters. Thousands did manage to escape, but thousands more are missing, without a trace, buried in a pile of rubble the size of a mountain.

The world is stunned. America is in shock, horrified by the death and destruction, terrified that the strongest nation in the world was caught off guard.

In a collective daze, we carry on. The children go to school. The adults make every effort to reassure themselves that the world will not come to an end. Government, in particular, displays a stiff upper lip. Legislative hearings go on as scheduled, as we get on with our lives.

In the State House, I visit with Senator Bev Hollingworth, a friend of my mother who is planning to run for governor.

"How's your mother doing?" Bev asks with genuine concern in her voice.

I tell her about Susie's approach to living in the moment, even as she lets go of the future and slips into the past. Bev tells me the story of her first marriage, raising four children after her husband was diagnosed with cancer.

"We lived every day as if it was our last day together," Bev says. "We traveled with our kids and talked about life. We appreciated the small things and didn't dwell on our problems. In the end, we became closer as a family."

Then Bev asks, "How's Malcolm holding up?"

I tell her Susie's quote about how kind Malcolm is to her now. Bev recalls their time sharing an office:

"Your mother seemed so powerful to me all day, negotiating deals in the Senate and getting her way. But every night at five-thirty, your father would call and I could hear her voice change on the phone. 'Yes dear, I'll meet you at the Holiday Inn to swim and then we'll go home for a delicious dinner.' She would get off the phone and say, 'Malcolm doesn't have any idea what I do all day, he just cares if I have dinner on the table.' I've always remembered that and wondered how she could manage her two separate lives."

☙

That evening I go home to help the boys with their homework and get dinner on the table. Travis, a fifth-grader, hasn't seen the images on television. His life is protected as he lies on the couch, reading *The Adventures of Huckleberry Finn*.

By contrast, Zach, an eighth-grader, has been talking about the terrorist attacks on New York and Washington all day long in school. In his engineering class, they discussed the construction of the towers and how the heat of the bomb blast melted the steel beams, causing the whole structure to collapse floor by floor. In English class, they were assigned an essay, "Where were you and what were you thinking when you heard the news?" Zach and his buddies have been talking about the draft, too.

Where did all these ideas come from? How did they come into our lives in just a day and a half?

On Friday morning, my friends and I gather at my house for our weekly yoga. With hugs all around and plenty of tears, we talk about the fear in our hearts and in our homes.

During yoga, my friend Anne begins to cry; she is missing her mother, who died years ago.

"Think of all those children losing their mothers and fathers," she says through her tears. The loss is overwhelming to us. We all need to hug our own mothers this week.

Lucia is sad because her mother is lost to Alzheimer's, alive but not available to comfort her. Beth is worried about her sister, who escaped from her office across from the World Trade Center but now is in shock.

After yoga, my friends Susan and Becky give me a birthday breakfast, but our spirits are low. Susan tells of a friend who escaped from his office building and ran through the streets of lower Manhattan to safety.

Becky wonders aloud how God could let this happen and whatever is the lesson to be learned from this tragedy? Sharing stories of courageous Americans saving the lives of strangers, I am reminded of my grandmother's lifelong lesson: "Be kind to all you meet." We are all suddenly aware that life is very short.

When I arrive at my mother's condo later on Friday morning, she is looking over a stack of photos.

"I can't remember anything. These pictures are rejects from my journal." My mother seems lost and confused.

"When you look at the pictures do you remember the trip?" I ask.

"I do remember the trip, but not these pictures," she explains I start the tape recorder. "Tell me what this is like for you." I say.

I feel like the rest of my life is over. I don't remember the present, those pictures, for instance. But I remember every one of those pictures all along there [she's pointing to the family pictures on the mantel again].

"When you woke up in the morning this week, did you remember about the attacks on New York and Washington?" I ask.

Yes, I did, because that was so important. But I can't remember what we did last weekend.

Not knowing what the answer will be, I ask quietly, "How does it make you feel? Is it sad or scary or frustrating?"

Well, for one thing, Daddy is very good about it. I feel that he has resented me in the past and now he's back to the beginning.

He married me because I was five years younger than he was. We went to England. I think that until I got to the legislature, he was superior. Then I became a feminist. I did all these things that were equal to him.

Now I'm going back to being nonequal to him and he appreciates that. He really is very kind and good about it. He hasn't always been good about the legislature and such. [She smiles.]

45

I am struck by her insight and her candor. "I had a wonderful visit with Bev Hollingworth the other day. She sends all her love to you. Do you remember Bev in the Senate? She's going to run for governor."

Susie responds, "Yes, I do remember her."

I told the story to my mother. "Bev was talking about when she shared an office with you in the Senate. Daddy wanted to go swimming every evening after work. Then he wanted to come home and have a nice dinner ready for him. She was talking about how your public persona was so powerful, so confident, so in charge. Remember when you were on the cover of the magazine as 'The Most Powerful Woman in New Hampshire'?" I ask.

My mother nods, smiling now, so I continue.

"Bev said it was so strange when Malcolm would call to say it was time to go for the swim. You would say, 'Okay, sweetie, I'll meet you there.' You would get off the phone and say, 'He doesn't have any idea what I'm doing all day long. I might be in a meeting. I might have something important to do.' Bev was remarking that you always would go. You didn't resist. You didn't say, 'I can't be there.' "

My mother looks delighted to hear this story.

It's just so marvelous that she said this. That's just how I felt. I felt very much inferior to him all along. That was the era.

"The role of women was changing, but you didn't want to cause conflict in your marriage. You wanted it to work out and not be threatening to him," I suggest. Susie nods, smiling.

Yes, that's just it.

In 1992, during her last session in the legislature, my mother was instrumental in forming a bipartisan coalition with the Senate Democrats to elect her friend Ralph Hough as Senate president. Although Susie was never assigned the title (so as not to offend the men in the Senate), she served as vice president of the Senate. Describing her role, my mother said,

Jeanne Shaheen and I would go up to Ralph's office at the end of the day to tell him what to do the next day in the Senate.

My mother is smiling now and her eyes are twinkling. She seems genuinely pleased that Bev and I understand what she was thinking at the time about balancing her role in the Senate with her role at home.

I feel weepy over that because Bev totally got it. To this day, I cook for him and love him, but in a way that's completely different from you. You're equal in a way that I never was.

Malcolm was a Rhodes scholar and I hadn't finished college. I was president of my freshman class. Then I left college because I got pregnant. I had an exam in the morning. I married him in the afternoon. I got an A on the exam. And that was it. I was inferior to him from then on. Now he realizes that I'm inferior to him and he's twice as kind.

"Even though I feel equal with my law degree and my job, it doesn't change the dynamic of taking care of the family," I reply. "I still get home at the end of the work day to cook dinner. Some things in the world have changed since your time and some things have not."

Susie is smiling as she says,

That's just it. You can spend money, but the money doesn't cook dinner!

"At least Brad does all the dishes," I say with a smile. "We do have a nice dinner together as a family. One doesn't have to be superior or inferior; we just want to be happy."

My mother and I are completely focused now on understanding each other's lives. In all the years juggling our work and family roles, we have never spoken so openly about our feelings. Slowly, we begin to realize that we share a dilemma. My mother and I want to make the world a better place, in our public and our private lives.

"I'm trying to understand how the role of women has changed and how your life might have been different. Say you had won when you ran for Congress. How would your life have been different?" I ask innocently.

I have said that I was running for Congress, but I couldn't feel more strongly that when I lost, I came home.

I never thought that I was going to win. . . . [She pauses, searching for the words.] *. . . If I had won, I think I would have gotten divorced.*

My mother's blunt response comes as no surprise. Her words remind me of a scene when she was running for Congress in 1980. She went off to campaign school in Washington. While she was there, she met with a group of Congresswomen. They all sat around in a circle with their shoes off and their feet up, because their feet were so sore in their high heels.

My mother told me later that all the Congresswomen were divorced or having trouble in their marriages. The women talked about how difficult campaigning and politics was on their husbands and their families. I wanted my mother to win the election and we campaigned hard throughout the summer, but I have never forgotten that scene.

I am reminded once again of the circular nature of my own thoughts about the changing role of women in Susie's world. All my life, I have been proud of my mother, both for her own political achievements and for her encouragement of women in politics.

My mother has dedicated her life to advancing the role of women by increasing the number of women elected to public office. She was an early member of the National Women's

Political Caucus, as well as a national board member of the Women's Campaign Fund and a strong supporter of Emily's List ("early money is like yeast," the key to a successful political campaign), raising money for progressive women candidates. Over the years, she raised more than $100,000 for the Women's Campaign Fund with annual lakeside luncheons to support progressive women candidates.

In 1992, Congresswoman Patricia Schroeder "tested the waters" at our home on Newfound Lake as she considered a bid in the New Hampshire presidential primary. In recent years, my mother has devoted her energy to The White House Project, aiming to elect a woman president of the United States. Her motto is "A woman's place is in the house — the State House and the White House!"

I share her strong conviction that women have a distinct and important role in shaping public policy. But as I look back on my life in Susie's world, I am more aware than most people would be of both the positive and the negative impact on the family of a political life. Women in politics need a wife, a daughter, a twin sister even, who can feed and nurture the family while the candidate is out making the world a better place.

For months now, Susie has been telling everyone, "Annie is my replacement." I indulge her with a gracious smile, knowing that for now, I'm balancing my life decisions with raising my own family. I don't want to miss the teen years this time around. I want to be present in the lives of my sons, my husband, my parents, and my friends. I don't want to miss our time together.

My mother has lived a life filled with color, brilliant, bright, dazzling and sometimes overwhelming. Having shared her with politics for more than thirty years, I appreciate our time together now. As we talk, I am learning how to make my way in my own life.

CHAPTER NINE

CHICKEN SOUP
FOR THE SUPREME SOUL

LATER DURING MY VISIT, my mother becomes visibly anxious and confused. "I want to send David Souter a birthday card," she explains, "but Malcolm was supposed to bring it to me." She wanders around her living room, searching for the card in piles of notes and invitations.

"No problem," I assure her. "I have a card that you can send to him."

She seems relieved and carefully writes out a birthday note. "I can hardly write anymore," she says. "But I don't want to miss David's birthday!"

One of the most difficult calls I had to make about my mother's decline was to Justice Souter in January 2001. She was going to Washington for her last national board meeting. I was anxious about my mother traveling alone, but I knew that she was excited to be visiting her good friends David Souter at the Supreme Court and Dave Broder at the *Washington Post*. I also knew that this would be her last trip traveling alone.

Although I was worried about my mother's safety, I was even more concerned about her loss of discretion and whether Justice Souter's trust in her confidentiality was now in jeopardy. I decided to call and give him fair warning.

"This is one of the hardest calls I've ever made," I began. "I know how much your friendship and your confidence over the years have meant to my mother." Then I told Justice Souter about my mother's loss of memory and discretion.

At first, he was undaunted, "Oh, Annie, don't worry."

But I persisted, "No, I am worried, about you and your privacy."

Then he understood and said, "Annie, this must be very hard for you. I appreciate your call." I hung up knowing that this call marked the end of an era.

჻

My mother and I settle in again by the fireplace as I begin taping. She is recalling how she came to be such a close friend and confidante to a U. S. Supreme Court justice. She begins telling me about her most recent visit from Justice Souter just a few weeks ago.

This last time, I gave him chicken soup that I had made myself. I sent him home with two containers of it because he just adored it. He went on and on about it. He ate the soup for lunch two days later.

I remember when David Souter was selected to be a Rhodes scholar. I was very proud of him. He came back from Oxford to Harvard Law School. Then he came to Malcolm's law office in Concord. He became assistant attorney general and then attorney general when I was in the legislature.

I was going to South Africa on a legislative trip, so I went to Washington a few days early for David's Supreme Court confirmation hearing. I sat right in the front row and loved every minute of it!

President Bush's chief of staff and our former governor, John Sununu, told the national press, "David Souter was a home run for the conservative right." The national women's groups started to gear up to fight the Souter nomination.

My mother knew better. On her own, she talked quietly behind the scenes with her friends in the women's movement about David Souter. Having served with him on the Concord Hospital Board for years, my mother knew his thinking on sensitive health issues. She believed that David Souter would uphold *Roe v. Wade*, supporting women's reproductive rights, including the right to freedom of choice.

The women's groups eventually backed down. The Souter nomination was confirmed by the Senate overwhelmingly. My mother was delighted.

I will always remember the evening in June 1992, as we sat around the dining room table at Newfound Lake with our good friends the Delanos, eating another of Susie's incredible meals. We toasted David Souter and his colleagues Sandra Day O'Connor and Anthony Kennedy, as I read aloud from the *Casey* decision, upholding *Roe v. Wade*:

> "An entire generation has come of age free to assume *Roe's* concept of liberty in defining the capacity of women to act in society, and to make reproductive decisions . . ."

The justices were writing about my generation. Without David Souter in the 5–4 majority in the *Casey* decision, *Roe v. Wade* could have been overturned. The Supreme Court ruling in *Casey* confirmed that men and women will continue to have the opportunity to plan their families and pursue their dreams.

Although my mother has no regrets about the decisions in her life, she knows that millions of Americans now "assume *Roe's* concept of liberty" in planning their lives. Without Justice Souter and his colleagues in the majority on the Supreme Court, this assumption and "the capacity of women to act in society" would be lost.

When President Clinton was inaugurated for his second term in January 1997, Justice Souter invited my mother to be his guest at the Supreme Court luncheon. When she arrived, Susie realized that she was Justice Souter's only guest. The other justices invited only their spouses.

She kissed Justice Souter at the door, and from then on she was his family. She sat with Justices Antonin Scalia and Clarence Thomas, holding forth in a lively conversation. Susie loved every minute, despite the fact that she rarely agrees with either one of them. On the way out, she kissed them all good-bye and they invited her back, anytime.

CHAPTER TEN

DISASTER RELIEF

ON FRIDAY EVENING, we gather with our friends at Beth's house for dinner. We crave community and connection. The children are relieved to hang out together and watch a movie. The adults relax, enjoying the company and conversation of close friends.

My friend Ellen asks how my parents are doing. I describe the contrast between my mother's approach to living in the moment and my father's focus on planning for the future or reminiscing about the past.

Ellen says with a smile, "One foot in the future, one foot in the past, and you're pissing on the present!"

We all agree that we are too shaken by the events of the week to think much about our past or our future. Tonight we are living in the moment.

Beth's dinner is delicious—harvest salad, roast chicken, and plenty of wine. Our conversation drifts from our global fears to raising our children. We are four professional couples who moved to this small town in New Hampshire to find peace and prosperity for our families. Doctors, lawyers, teachers, and social workers, each of us is searching for a safe environment in which to raise our children.

Our generation of parents has been obsessed for years with breast feeding our babies, childproofing our homes, and buying sporting helmets of every shape and kind. Now we are entering a new era.

Our teenagers face risks that we all remember. My parents' generation simply looked the other way. In my mother's words, describing me at age twelve, "You were all grown. The independence from me was a good thing."

Around the dinner table tonight we have stories of friends who made it through the teen years intact, and of those who did not. The question we face is, How do we raise thoughtful, compassionate, careful children in a world full of risk?

As we are leaving, each child lights a candle. We stand in a circle singing patriotic songs. Tonight we are joined in our sorrow for the victims and in our pride for the heroes. Through our tears, we sing of the "land of the free and the home of the brave," with each child's face shining in candlelight.

୬

Saturday morning, Zach and I wake up early to drive to his soccer game in Exeter. We listen to National Public Radio about the horrors of the day. Zach sits quietly, taking it all in. Then he asks, "Mom, if a nuclear bomb drops on Washington, where is the government after that?"

"I don't know the answer, Zach. I suppose there is a contingency plan somewhere. But I wish you didn't have to ask the question," I say with tears in my eyes.

Scott Simon is hosting a call-in show about the U.S. response to the terrorist attack. One woman describes her view that "the world should embrace peace in the new millennium and seek a higher world order based upon spiritual growth and understanding."

His voice filled with emotion, Scott Simon responds, "I am from the Vietnam era and I support peace and justice, too. But I'm struggling because, although I don't want us to bomb innocent civilians in Afghanistan any more than you do, I don't want to see this happen in our country ever again." Zach and I share his view and his struggle.

After Zach's soccer game, I drive to Travis's game. En route, I call friends in New York and Washington to check in.

Laura, in Manhattan, is solemn. Her friends and family are safe, but she is feeling helpless and sad for her city.

"Laura, go back to work," I suggest. "Do your massage. Your magic fingers will ease the sorrow and heal the pain that people are feeling."

Nini, in Washington, is even more distressed. Nini and I worked together on Capitol Hill twenty years ago. She has lived and worked in Washington ever since. Now Nini knows too much about the terrorist attacks from her friends who work in the White House and on Capitol Hill. I'm trying to comprehend Nini's fear about terrorist cells in America, but the day is too perfect here in New Hampshire. I can't imagine her message in my reality.

"There are humvees in the streets and F-16's flying overhead all the time. This isn't the end, Annie, this is just the beginning," she says.

Fear settles into my skin. "I love you, Nini, I love you," I say when we hang up.

Then I talk with my oldest sister, Robin, whose daughter, Marion, was just beginning her first year of college at

Georgetown this week. Marion could see the Pentagon burning from her dormitory. I am relieved that Marion is safe on the Georgetown campus and meeting new friends.

Robin is pleased to hear about my visits with Susie. She laughs when I say that Susie was worried about whether Robin knew that she was pregnant when she got married.

"I didn't know until my boyfriend told me in college." She says, "I would love to hear more." I urge Robin to spend time with Susie now while they can both enjoy their time together.

At Travis's soccer game, the sky is deep blue and crystal clear, without a cloud or a plane in sight. The terror in our hearts and the peace of the day cannot be reconciled. Before the game begins, the referee lines up both teams. We have a moment of silence for the victims and their families. Then the boys play soccer and life goes on, one goal at a time.

అ

Saturday night, Brad and I go to a lovely inn on a lake for a gourmet dinner to celebrate our fifteenth wedding anniversary. We are not in a festive mood, but the food is exquisite and we appreciate our time together.

We talk about the flags on every house and the events of the week. Brad is concerned about the saber rattling, but I find comfort in the universal experience of grief. I tell him Susie's thoughts on living in the moment and coming to the end of her life. We feel vulnerable in our lives, but safe in our hearts.

That night I dream about the end of the world. I am frantically trying to count the mattresses in the bunker to be certain we have enough beds for our family. In the morning, I contemplate living a different life, filled with fear and plans to protect my family. I make crêpes for breakfast and take a hot tub in the sun, hoping the peace of the day will settle back into my bones.

As the morning passes, I realize that the only change I will make in my life is to live every moment to the fullest, knowing that it may be my last. I will set aside petty differences with my children, my husband, my friends and colleagues. I will live like my mother, in the present, with an open heart. There will be no strangers, just folks I haven't met yet. I will let the memory of misery fade first. By midday, I begin to feel the peace settle back into my heart.

ॐ

On Sunday afternoon, my parents come out to Hopkinton to watch Zach and Travis play soccer. The day is crystal clear and sunny again, with hawks soaring in the skies above where planes once flew. Susie settles in on the sidelines next to her dear old friend Betty, whose grandsons are playing soccer today, too.

Susie and Betty have led parallel lives for almost fifty years, raising large families in Concord since the late 1950s. Betty's oldest daughter, Lisa, has been my best friend since the third grade. All three of Betty's daughters are raising their families in Hopkinton, their children going to school and playing soccer with my boys.

Our conversation inevitably turns to the horrific events of the week and our fears about the future for our children and grandchildren. Susie and Betty recall the Cold War scares of the early 1960s. We are all reminded of the "duck-and-cover" drills in school and the bomb shelters.

I remember our neighbors building an underground bomb shelter, stocked with canned goods and cots. At age six, I was shocked to learn from a young friend next door that our large family would not be invited into the neighbor's bomb shelter. Memories that seemed quaint a week ago feel alarmingly real today.

Susie participates in the conversation as the topic ranges from building bomb shelters to the majestic hawks circling overhead in the brilliant blue sky. But when she tries to share her *New York Times,* Susie cannot recall Betty's name. A fifty-year friendship is now reduced to "that nice lady at the soccer game who wants to read my paper."

Monday is Travis's tenth birthday. My parents arrive with steak for dinner. We are all trying desperately to resume our lives. While I grill the steaks, we listen to the day's news, including the stock market crash and the Pakistani envoy to Afghanistan to capture Osama Bin Laden. Susie listens closely, but she is confused. "Did the stock market go way up today?" she asks.

During dinner, my mother hardly speaks at all, except to say from time to time, "This is marvelous, just marvelous." She takes pictures of Travis opening his presents and blowing out the candles on his cake. Whether it's the Alzheimer's or the events of last Tuesday, I'm aware that these innocent times together are rare and very precious.

On Tuesday, I find a glimmer of hope in the mailbox. Our friend Georgia Delano has sent a postcard from Manhattan. Georgia and Bill watched the horror unfold at the World Trade Center from their roof garden on East 10th Street. When their neighborhood was blocked off, they left the city by train, then borrowed a car to drive to New Hampshire. After a week of relative peace in the country, they are back home, caring for their city.

Georgia ends the postcard with a hopeful message, "p.s. Laura is a volunteer now, giving massages to the firefighters!" For the first time in a week, I cry tears of joy.

CHAPTER ELEVEN

THE THIRD FRIDAY:
PUBLIC SERVANT

THE RAIN COMES during the night. By Friday morning, the whole world is weeping. Two weeks of brilliant blue September skies finally give way to a downpour.

When I arrive at my mother's condo, I can tell that she's feeling blue, too. I have rarely seen my mother in a low mood. As I begin taping, I ask softly, "Tell me how you're feeling, Momma."

I'm feeling a little badly because I can't remember anything anymore. I feel for the first time that I really have Alzheimer's and . . . [she pauses, searching for the words] . . . that I can't talk anymore.

I went yesterday with Richard [Moore] down to Audubon in Manchester. It was a party at lunch. Malcolm was out to lunch. I didn't have to feed him, so I went. For the first time, I really got the sense that I couldn't speak.

On the way back in the car, I got the money for the tolls. That was very special to Richard, who was driving, but it was the only thing I did all day long that was significant. I really feel as though I hadn't done anything about the day. I was in charge of the fund-raising in the beginning, . . . but I don't feel that I could go to anybody anymore and talk.

Just a few years ago, my mother was president of the Audubon Society of New Hampshire. Her leadership and charm were key ingredients to the successful multimillion-dollar capital campaign to build the new nature center in Manchester. Yet today, her greatest achievement was finding the correct change for the tollbooth. Times have definitely changed.

So I just feel differently than I did . . . as long as I don't know people. I said on the phone today to the guy that was calling . . . [she pauses, searching for the words]. . . I can't even remember what it was about . . . it's going to be a thing next week in the legislature. I said "I can't go to the legislature anymore."

"That's the first time you've said that?" I ask.

Yes. He wanted me to come testify. I said that I couldn't go to the State House anymore.

"That is a big change," I say.

That really is. It happened today and yesterday. Malcolm is so worried about me because he is leaving for the weekend. He is going on an AMC board retreat and canoe trip. He said to me several times that he was worried about me driving down to Portsmouth to stay with Robin for the weekend.

I am pleased that my father is getting away for the weekend with the Appalachian Mountain Club Board. I am happy that Robin will have time alone with Susie. But now I'm beginning to worry.

"Do you think you can find Robin's house?" I ask.

Yes, I can. [She replies with confidence.] *Malcolm instructed me three times about how to get there.*

"Does it make you sad to think about this change?" I ask. "How do you feel about it?"

Well, I denied it for so long and now . . . [she pauses, as if she is distracted]. *. . . The taste of food is terrible. Cooking is just . . . I cook for him but not for myself at all.*

I am intrigued that my mother often connects her gradual decline with the loss of her sense of taste. We have learned that neurological changes in the front of the brain ultimately result in loss of taste and loss of memory. I remember, during our first medical appointment, that the neurologist suggested a simple test for Alzheimer's.

First, has the patient lost her sense of smell or taste? Second, has the patient ever found herself somewhere and not known how she got there? My mother lost her sense of taste several years ago, but she has never become so confused that she didn't know how she'd gotten somewhere.

Knowing what we know now about Susie's experience with Alzheimer's, the second part of the test seems cruel and outdated. In years past, the medical community was unwilling to acknowledge Alzheimer's disease until the patient was so confused that she did not know where she was or how she got there. No wonder patients became frustrated or even hostile when everyone was in denial until it was too late to care.

๛

Curious to know more about Susie's reaction to the recent changes in her life, I ask, "What did the doctor say at the last appointment?"

That I have Alzheimer's. . . . What I mean to do is call [she pauses again] *. . . I don't even remember her name.*

"Ellen Sheridan?" I ask, assuming that she means our family friend who is involved with the Alzheimer's Association. Ellen recently came to visit my parents to talk about their future. "She's our old friend who lived across the street," I begin to explain.

Well, I remember all of that back then. But I want to call her again to find out more about Alzheimer's.

"Ellen wants to help you, Mom. We'll give her a call. We will be here for you too," I reassure her. I want my mother to feel loved and to feel meaningful again in the world.

"Momma, do you want to do the taping now, before you forget anymore?" I ask.

Yes, let's do. [She smiles.]

"Let's pick up where you left off talking about the League of Women Voters and running for the legislature," I suggest. Susie smiles at me, looks at the tape recorder, and begins.

I was president of the auxiliary at the state hospital. We used to give a birthday party for the patients once a month. I lit the candles on the cake but nobody came.

It turned out that the hospital had a rule that patients couldn't get out of bed unless there were clean sheets when they returned. They were saving money by not doing laundry. So they kept them in bed waiting for the laundry, while the birthday candles went out.

I was so upset. I went home and told Malcolm that I was

going to run for the legislature because I wanted to fix the tax structure of the State of New Hampshire.

There were three thousand patients in the state mental hospital in the 1960s. I remember walking with my mother through the wards, metal beds filled with patients rocking, moaning, and crying out. My mother volunteered in the hospitality shop. She organized square dances and a birthday party every month for the patients.

One of the crowning achievements of my mother's legislative career was passage of the law mandating insurance coverage for mental health. Ultimately, this law led to privately funded care for the mentally ill at the local level across New Hampshire. Meanwhile, advances in prescription medication and therapy provided hope for better mental health treatment.

Thousands of patients were sent home from the state hospital to live and work in their communities. New Hampshire now has one of the most advanced mental health delivery systems in the nation, with local mental health centers around the state and only a few hundred acute care patients in Concord. My mother is duly proud of her role in this achievement.

Wondering how she felt when her twenty-five-year legislative career first began, I ask, "How did you campaign the first time you ran?"

I didn't dare go door-to-door the first time, so I lost. But two years later, in 1969, I was braver. I stood on the court-house steps on Election Day on crutches because I had broken my foot dancing. It worked and I won!

Then my mother launches back onto the subject of her eternal quest to change the tax structure of the State of New Hampshire.

I studied a broad-based tax in the League of Women Voters. The Concord schools needed more support, but the property tax was too high. Our tax structure was "beer, butts, booze, bets, beds and bellies" . . . And that was it! . . . So I ran for the legislature to get a broad-based tax. I worked at it for twenty-five years and never got one.

New Hampshire is the only state in the union that has never had a broad-based tax. Alaska had a sales tax until they discovered oil. About ten years ago, New Jersey was the next to last state. The Hager-Below income tax bill now is just incredible. But it's not going to pass.

Yesterday in the newspaper I read about the president of the Senate and the speaker of the house opposing the income tax. They think the solution is "more beer, butts, booze, bets, beds, and bellies"!

Despite her memory loss, my mother still has vivid recollections of her experiences in the State House. "What was it like for women in the legislature back then?" I ask.

I remember that the women were better than the men in the legislature. They all came out of the League of Women Voters. The men were not the types that could earn money. They were the types that couldn't.

There were 400 members and 89 women when I was there and it grew to 125 women. It was the women that inspired me. I became a feminist when I turned 40 and I wasn't up until then.

I became convinced that government needs more women. The women worked hard and studied the issues. I did a study of the men and women getting out of their cars in the morning. The women changed into high heels and grabbed a huge load of books, papers, and mail. The men put on their jackets and ties and walked into the State House empty-handed.

"How did you get along with the other legislators and work effectively with them for so many years?" I wonder aloud.

When I ran for speaker of the house, I went to see 206 legislators in their homes. That was an experience in itself that was really vital to understanding them and working with them.

One guy was in his barn about to deliver a calf. He wrapped a rope around its feet. As he pulled, he said, "If it's a heifer, I'll vote for you!" Out came a huge calf. When he lifted its leg, he said, "It's a George (the name of the man I was running against), but I'm taking him to be turned into veal tomorrow!"

I came to realize that the women discussed the issues and the men didn't discuss the issues at all. I was a good friend of the majority leader. (I can't remember his name.) It was interesting to get what you wanted without sleeping with the men, which is what several women did in the legislature! [She laughs.]

Once again, my mother's candor is disarming, yet charming. Her words distill twenty-five years of her life experience, focusing on the highlights.

I'm curious about the evolution of her party politics. "How did your party affiliation change over the years?" I ask.

For fifty-five years, I was a Republican. I gave the first party for George Bush when he ran for president in the New Hampshire presidential primary. Our house was so wonderful. His people came to ask me if we would give a party.

I was so enthusiastic about George Bush and I knew Barbara very well from the campaign, so I said yes. I cooked all the food. George Bush couldn't believe that I made the hors d'oeuvres and the dinner all by myself. I gave a good party!

When I retired after twenty-five years in the Legislature and Malcolm retired from his law firm, we took a trip around the world. My friend Liz Hager ran for my seat in the State Senate.

When Liz lost in the Republican primary, we switched to Democrat. Malcolm said he would have done it twelve years before if it hadn't been for me. I taped a radio ad for the Democrat, Sylvia Larsen, over the telephone from Kuala Lumpur. Sylvia won my seat. We've been Democrats ever since!

I wrote an op-ed piece that was published in the New York Times *comparing my life with Barbara Bush, called "Barbara and Me." We both married war heroes and raised five children. We look alike, too, with our white hair and pearls! Both George Bush and Barbara stayed with us during the New Hampshire primary. She even wore my bathing suit for a swim in Newfound Lake when the advance man lost her luggage.*

Barbara remained the loyal politician's wife, but I became a feminist in the New Hampshire Legislature. I was pro-choice and George Bush wasn't anymore. I wrote in the New York Times *that I was voting for Bill Clinton for president!*

Then I met Hillary Clinton. I will never forget introducing her for a speech in Washington. She is perfect!

As we wind down our taping for the day, I am impressed once again by my mother's life experience and her candor. I have come to appreciate a certain trade-off in this stage of her life. Although she might have remembered more details if we had taped her story a year ago, she is so much more direct now. Alzheimer's has removed her discretionary filter. Susie is Susie, nothing more, but not a whole lot less.

CHAPTER TWELVE

The Fourth Friday: 'Crown Thy Good with Sisterhood'

FRIDAY NIGHT IS Travis's birthday party with his whole soccer team. The party is a wild affair, with fifteen ten-year-old boys playing soccer and flashlight tag into the night. We serve pizza and birthday cake. As the boys pile into the vans for the ride home, everyone agrees that "this is the best party we've ever been to. We just wish it could have lasted longer!"

Birthday parties were a big deal when I was growing up. In a big family, each child is the star for one special day. Susie would organize fun parties, with hats and birthday cake in the backyard or hiking and hot dogs over the fire out in the country.

One year, Robin worked hard and saved her money to buy a bike. Then Donald scheduled his birthday party on a Sunday and told his friends to just bring a dollar instead of buying a present. Donald had his bike in a day, and Robin never forgave him.

༺༻

Saturday morning, we drive up to Newfound Lake to take our boat out of the water. The day is glorious again, unseasonably warm with clear skies. American flags adorn every house, mailbox, and pickup truck. Patriotic fervor merges with sympathy for the victims and their families.

The trees are beginning to turn up north. Brilliant reds and bright yellows line the lake, as the sun sparkles on the deep blue water.

My aunt Lilla arrives at the house just as we pull into the driveway. She asks how my mother is doing and how my father is managing. After all these years, Lilla is still Malcolm's protective older sister.

Over the summer, Lilla learned how to give Susie time to talk, without finishing her sentences or interrupting. This is a challenge for McLanes, who are born talkers. Lilla is delighted that my "Fridays with Susie" are a success. She is intrigued to hear Susie's reaction to her fate with Alzheimer's.

At age eighty, my aunt Lilla has led a long and productive life. She is full of energy and enthusiasm for a wide range of charitable causes. Lilla raised six children in Hanover. Now she lives at Kendal and continues to work hard every day to make the world a better place.

My aunt Lilla was the first person I called to help create the Women's Fund of New Hampshire. When she said, "I'm not into women's issues," I said, "Lilla, I'm just asking for your wisdom for one year." She became a founding member of the board and a convert to our cause. We raised more than $2.5 million in three years to create an endowment to benefit the lives of women and girls in New Hampshire. Lilla was key to our success.

As we sit by the lake, Lilla opens her heart with the story of her emotional breakdown when she turned fifty and her children were almost all grown. "I was the chair of the board at the mental health center, so they treated me well," my aunt says with a smile. "I realized then that I needed to help other people, to make a difference in the world."

Lilla found meaning in her life by creating a better world for those in need. She served on boards and raised money for dozens of social service agencies. Generations of Dartmouth students have worked with Lilla, volunteering to build a house for Habitat for Humanity or grow organic food for low-income families in the Upper Valley. No cause is too small, no problem is too big for my aunt to rise to the challenge. Both Lilla and Susie have done well in the world by doing good for others. I am inspired by the choices they have made, by the decisions that have shaped their lives.

༄

Friday morning is Susie's seventy-second birthday. When we call to sing her "Happy Birthday," Susie is pleased to report that the *Concord Monitor* remembered, too. "This day in New Hampshire history" reads:

> "**1929** Susan McLane is born. She will serve as a state senator for Concord after also representing the city in the House. She will run unsuccessfully for Congress, just losing out in the primary to Judd Gregg."

Later in the day, I arrive at my parents' house with my mother's birthday cake and gift. Her older sister, Mary, and my uncle Bob Kilmarx are here for Susie's birthday lunch. Mary recently retired from a successful career in energy policy in

Rhode Island. Both in their seventies, Mary and Bob seem to defy aging, playing tennis weekly year-round and sailing their own boat to Maine every summer.

Mary and Bob share photos of their walking tour of the Cotswolds in England. My mother sits quietly as we engage in a lively conversation.

Mary and Bob want to hear about my Fridays with Susie. They are pleased to hear that our time together is successful. I realize that today my mother cannot get a word in edgewise, but when I talk about recording her life story, Susie says with a smile, "I am so flattered!"

My father tells about Susie's trip to Portsmouth last weekend. She did get lost, both arriving and leaving, but her problem-solving skills were fully intact. Susie found the chamber of commerce for a map to find Robin's house and a policeman for directions to find her way home.

"Once I was on the highway, I had no problem," my mother says proudly. We all agree that Susie needs Malcolm as her navigator and that she will not drive alone outside of Concord anymore.

Coping with Alzheimer's is like raising a child, only in reverse. The changes are subtle, but every once in a while we realize that Susie cannot do something that seemed simple just a few weeks ago. Her birthday party is a jolly occasion, but I know that the next time we are all together, Susie will have slipped even further away.

CHAPTER THIRTEEN

'Try to Remember That Day in September'

October arrives with a cold snap. The temperature drops in the night, and by morning the last of the petunias wilt from the frost. The boys finally wear long pants to school. I pull out my first turtleneck of the season, apple green to brighten my day.

The day is beautiful, but not perfect. At five minutes to four, I realize that I have locked my keys in the car. Damn, I'm going to be late to the dentist. Anxiously searching my purse for the keys, then spotting them inside the car, my first reaction is anger and frustration. I can't find the spare key under the bumper, so I call Brad for a ride, only to reach his voice mail. I'm frantic.

Then I pause, take a deep breath, and think of my mother. Three children under age five, two broken legs, and pregnant on crutches with her fourth. *"And so . . . there it was."* Five children under eight, with three in diapers at the same time, and no car all day. *"And so . . . there it was."* What was I worried about anyway?

Suddenly, the day feels sunny and warm, the leaves are starting to turn. The walk up the hill to the dentist feels good. I won't be on time, but life will go on. Besides, the exercise is good for me. Arriving ten minutes later, I sink into the dentist's chair with a smile. Life could be worse, much worse.

What caused me to leave my keys in the car? I was rushing to a partners meeting at 7:30 in the morning. I woke up early, quietly took a hot bath, drank my coffee, and glanced through the stack of mail and newspapers on the kitchen counter. When the boys woke up, I made their cinnamon toast, served their breakfast, made Travis's lunch, got dressed, dried my hair, brushed my teeth, kissed everyone good-bye, and ran out the door. I parked on the street so I wouldn't be late to the meeting. I remembered to feed the meter but apparently forgot my keys in the car.

Later in the morning, as I buried myself in e-mails and telephone calls from clients, I forgot to move my car to the parking garage. When I found the car with the keys inside, there were two tickets on the windshield. Then, in my frustration over the keys, I forgot to feed the meter. When Brad picked me up at the dentist and brought me back to unlock my car, I found another parking ticket. Even my mother's optimism cannot brighten this day!

I begin to wonder: Is my life too crazy or is my mother's Alzheimer's disease becoming contagious? What happens when our brain reaches its limit of function?

৵

On Wednesday morning, I call my parents to wish my father a happy birthday. My mother answers and we talk for several minutes. My father has left for the office. After fifty years of a distinguished career as a trusts and estates lawyer, Malcolm goes each morning to the firm to read his mail and pick up the *New York Times*. He appreciates the time in town and Susie is happy to putter around the house on her own.

This morning, my mother is trying to tell me what they have been doing, but she cannot find the words. I wait patiently to let her express her thoughts, but the words are simply not there. Finally, I try to help. "Did you go out to dinner for Daddy's birthday?" I ask.

"No, that's tonight. We are going up to the lake for lunch today. Then tonight we are going out to dinner." [She pauses, then tries again.] *"We got up early this morning . . . then we drove there . . . before he went to the office . . .* [Another pause, and then finally she finds the word.] *. . . to the recycling place. We took all the cans and bottles and papers from the garage."*

She sounds pleased with herself. We talk a bit longer about their day and whether I should come out for a birthday lunch.

"Call my husband to make the plan," my mother says. She pauses, "I'm having trouble talking this morning."

Now my mother sounds sad and confused.

"No problem, Momma. I'll call Daddy right now. I'll see you soon. I love you." I say softly.

I am sad, too, when I hang up, knowing that Susie can feel herself slipping away, knowing that she knows, too.

When I call my father, he also stays on the line. We talk for fifteen minutes, the longest I have ever talked with him on the phone. My parents are leaving for the lake this morning, so I make plans to come out to their house for a visit on Friday.

Then we discuss my mother, her decline and how they're coping. I tell my father what my mother said over the past few weeks about not going to any more meetings and not being able to talk with people she does not know well. He is well aware of these changes, noting that she often comments after a visit with friends, "I didn't talk at all."

The two of them, however, are doing just fine together. My father mentions their new plan to visit Marion in Washington and drive to the Eastern Shore to stay with new friends from their trip to Alaska. He tells me about their dinner last night eating lobsters with their friend Priscilla. "Susie was just fine, enjoying every minute!" he insists.

My father is changing, too. He is still making plenty of plans for the future, but now he is living more in the moment. Every day my parents plan something to do—driving to the lake, going out to lunch, or meeting friends for dinner. My father knows this time with my mother is precious and that it will not last forever. He appreciates their long, slow dance together.

෴

For my father's birthday, I have bought a new book on Alzheimer's disease, *The Forgetting*, by David Shenk. In keeping with our family tradition, I read it first before giving it away. Since my father's mother had Alzheimer's in the 1970s, the number of Americans afflicted has risen from 500,000 to more than five million. As the baby boomers become seniors, that number will climb to fifteen million.

Shenk explains that more and more people realize now what is happening to them at an earlier stage in the progression. He talks about how people will react with greater knowledge of the disease but no cure and not much in the way of treatment:

> *What will they do with the advance knowledge? It is not an easy question. Will they use the time left to get their affairs in order and to prepare themselves emotionally for the long fade? Or will the knowledge only add to the frustration and*

force them into a psychological spiral to accompany the physiological one?

Thus far in our journey, my mother is inclined toward using the time left to get her affairs in order and to prepare herself emotionally for "the long fade." When I asked her recently if she was worried about her future, she said with supreme confidence, "No, I have read about Alzheimer's. The thing about Alzheimer's is that you don't think about the future. So, you don't worry about the future."

When my mother said these words, I realized that I could let go of my worries, too. Rather than dwell on the future and let the frustration force us into a "psychological spiral to accompany the physiological one," I will live with her in the moment, appreciating the quality of our life together. Our time together will be her parting gift to me. Capturing her story will be my parting gift to her. We will savor our last dance together.

CHAPTER FOURTEEN

THE FIFTH FRIDAY: PRIMARY CARE

WHEN I ARRIVE at my mother's condo on Friday morning, I am once again remembering my mother's mother, who loved to remind us all that patience is a virtue, to which my mother would reply:

> *Patience is a virtue,*
> *Possess it if you can,*
> *Seldom found in woman,*
> *Never found in man!*

I am thinking about patience and the precious nature of our time together. No matter how hectic my life becomes during the week, juggling client meetings, legislative hearings, dentist appointments, charitable commitments, and soccer practices with meals, laundry, homework, and meaningful time with my family,

I feel at peace as soon as I walk through my mother's door each Friday morning.

Today when I begin taping, Susie is at a loss for words.

I can't talk anymore. I just feel as though I have deteriorated so in the last week or two.

Concerned about her decline, I ask my mother about her doctor and the medicine she is taking now.

It's the female doctor in Concord. I like her a lot. I have the bottle of medicine, but you have to come see it. [She takes me into her bathroom and shows me an entire medicine cabinet of various vials.]

"You were on Aricept before, but now you have switched to Exelon," I explain. My mother cannot comprehend the names of the various prescriptions, although she does realize that the medicine has been helpful.

Then Susie brings out a new book, *Alzheimer's: Loss of Self,* to share with me. We begin talking about the gradual onset of Alzheimer's and how her life has changed over the past eighteen months.

"You and I went to the doctor in the spring a year and a half ago. He said 'you don't have Alzheimer's. You had a stroke. Take one aspirin a day,' " I recount as my mother listens attentively.

"Then last summer, up until your birthday, we thought that was just it. But by last fall and winter, things started to get worse. Eventually, you started taking Aricept," I say as I try to piece together the timeline of her decline.

Yeah, that's it. [She nods, smiling.]

"Then somebody took you off the Aricept," I add. While I was staying with my parents in February recovering from knee surgery, I realized that my mother was declining day by day. When I expressed my concern to my father, he said that during the last visit, the doctor had asked her whether she thought the medicine was working. When she said, "I don't know," the doctor took her off the medicine.

I remember thinking, Why would a doctor ask a woman with Alzheimer's disease who takes a dozen medications a day whether she thought one of them was working? A health care client of mine told me about Aricept, so I mentioned it to my father. He checked the vial in the trash and reported that it was the Aricept that the doctor had discontinued.

"Apparently, it was working just fine for her. Are there any refills left?" I asked.

"Yes, and I'm going right down to the pharmacy to fill the prescription and get her back on it," my father said, sounding hopeful.

After that incident with the neurologist, my mother went back to her primary care physician. She is fond of her own woman doctor, Tanya Vanderlinde. Dr. Vanderlinde switched my mother's medication to Exelon, the most recent to emerge among two dozen Alzheimer's medicines now in the research-and-development stage.

Now in the last week I just can't find the words. I'm going to the doctor in November and I can't wait. I just want to talk with the doctor about it.

"What's so hard for everybody is that maybe the doctor can't do anything for you. Maybe Tanya can't help us." I am cautious as I explain to my mother, "They keep talking about a cure for Alzheimer's or a treatment, but I think these are the only two prescription medicines that are available now."

I am trying to balance reality with hope. I want to match my mother's candor without breaking her heart, or mine.

I just feel so strongly that more people are getting Alzheimer's all the time. [She smiles.]

In recent months, Alzheimer's has been the cover story in *Time* magazine. Everyone is suddenly talking about the Alzheimer's "epidemic." According to *Time*, "On average, 10% of people over age 65 come down with Alzheimer's, a number that rises to 50% by age 85." Given the aging population in America and throughout the world, a growing number of people and their families will soon be coping with the disease.

"What would you tell people about how to cope with Alzheimer's?" I ask innocently.

Well, that I don't want to live anymore. That is principally it. I am willing to die tomorrow. (That is very private. I can't say that and I don't tell that to Malcolm, at all.)

I've led a really good life. You are my replacement in life. This story makes me teary because you are so wonderful.

I am amazed once again by my mother's frankness and composure.

"I think it's an important story, Momma. It's worthwhile for people, both the life that you led and the life you're still leading. You could help all those people trying to cope with Alzheimer's and all their families, too," I say, trying to reassure my mother and myself.

Making life more meaningful for people with Alzheimer's, and helping their families cope with the loss, will be my mother's lasting contribution to the world, her final encore.

I am trying hard to be compassionate, yet stay rational. This moment is the essence of my mother's experience with Alzheimer's. She has led a good life, a productive life, a meaningful life. Now she is "willing to die tomorrow."

My mother is able to let go because she is planning to pass on the torch to me. I realize now that the central questions in my life are whether I am willing to let her go and whether I am able to accept the torch.

I am reminded of the innocent victims of the terrorist attacks calling their loved ones on cell phones from the World Trade Towers and the hijacked airplanes to say "I love you . . . good-bye." For the people about to die, these calls may have provided peace of mind. But those on the receiving end are bewildered, left to cope with the loss and to carry on.

For years, I have known that my mother would be a tough act to follow. When she retired from the legislature in 1994, I considered running for her State Senate seat. My boys were then only three and six years old. I remember thinking at the time that my life might be more flexible and manageable serving in the legislature than practicing law.

In the end, the most influential people in my life—my husband, my parents, and my boss—all thought I would be crazy to give up a successful law practice to serve in the legislature for two hundred dollars every two years. Faced with the reality of college savings, retirement planning, and all the expenses of a growing family, I decided not to run.

In hindsight, it was the right decision for our family. My law practice developed into lobbying on behalf of colleges and health care providers, so I still get my public policy fix. Like skiing, politics is in our genes.

ふ

Now my mother's life is changing, in subtle and sometimes mysterious ways. When I ask for her advice about coping with the disease, she replies:

How to cope with Alzheimer's? . . . Well, I don't sleep very well. About every third night I take a strong sleeping pill. I take two at the lake when I'm sleeping with Malcolm.

I venture back to the most difficult question: "When you say you are willing to die tomorrow, is there a part of you that might even prefer that to a long, slow decline?"

"Yes that's just it."

Our eyes lock onto each other. I feel closer to my mother in this moment than ever before in my life.

"I think that's the way I've always thought about it," I say through my tears. "I've often wondered who would come to the church and what we would say at your memorial service. Now I think, maybe we won't get the chance to honor you in that way. Instead maybe the end of your life will be a long, slow decline.

"People ask me about you every day, all the time," I say. We are both smiling now. My mother looks proud.

"Do you remember Karen Wadsworth in the legislature? She told me a story yesterday from 1980 during your campaign for Congress when she was the mayor of Lebanon. We went to her house for an event. After the guests left, there was a terrible thunder and lightning storm. Karen was frightened and afraid to be alone. You stayed with her. You let your whole campaign schedule go, just to be with her. Karen told me, with tears in her eyes, 'That's the kind of person your mother was.' "

My mother looks pleased, but bewildered.

Oh, that's wonderful. But I don't remember it, at all! [She laughs.]

"Well, she thinks fondly of you," I say, laughing along with my mother. "Do you remember anything about your campaign for Congress?"

I remember that Hilary Cleveland (the wife of the congressman who had served for twenty years) called to say that she had two things to tell me. First, she asked if I would be the speaker at the Colby-Sawyer College graduation. Then she told me that Jim was not running again for Congress.

The legend is that Susie was standing in the kitchen in her nightgown. She got off the phone and turned to ask Malcolm if she could run for Congress.

"Of course. You don't have to ask me," he replied. "But you'll have to get dressed first!"

My mother then tells her favorite story from her congressional campaign.

> You and I were campaigning all over New Hampshire. One day, an old guy in a gas station said, "Lady, you should be home taking care of your babies." And I said, pointing at you filling up the tank, "That's my baby and she's taking care of me!"

We both laugh again. "We did spend a lot of time together that summer, driving fourteen thousand miles on the campaign trail," I recall fondly.

Susie and I share another favorite story from the campaign. My father's mother was eighty-nine years old with Alzheimer's at the time. Whenever we came to visit, my grandmother would ask my mother what she was doing and Susie would announce the big news that she was running for Congress.

My grandmother's enthusiastic response was always the same. "Wonderful! I'm proud of you. My mother [a leading New Hampshire suffragette] would be proud of you too! Can I give you any money for your campaign?"

Toward the end of the campaign, Susie would seek out my grandmother to tell her the big news over and over again. She always had the perfect reaction.

I was proud of my mother, too. "I can remember so clearly your speech to the Claremont Rotary Club, before there even were women in Rotary," I tell her now. "They all looked so surprised to have a woman talking about missile defense." Susie looks proud of the memory.

"We watched all the debates, you and nine men standing up on the stage. You would put on your jacket and step right up to speak your mind. Do you remember how that felt?" I wonder what Susie was thinking back then.

Yeah, I do. I beat Charlie Bass and I didn't lose to Judd Gregg by very much. [She pauses.]

Well, I didn't ever think I was going to get elected. That was when I first felt dissatisfied with the Republican Party. I can remember how incredible my daughters all were about the campaign. They kept me at it.

I felt that I was inferior in a way that my daughters don't feel. That was the era back then. Malcolm was ambivalent about me running for Congress. But I had a good time.

My mother came in second in the Republican primary, beating eight men and narrowly losing to Judd Gregg, who went on to serve as our congressman and then our U. S. Senator. She beat Charlie Bass, who later joined her in the New Hampshire Senate and eventually became our congressman.

We talk about Al Rock, a state senator who owned a radio station in southern New Hampshire. He was a conservative Republican who opposed my mother. We bought several weeks of radio ads on his station, but the ads were never broadcast.

Susie ran well across the district except in the southern tier. For years, we wondered whether those radio ads might have made any difference.

He never played my ads. He paid me back the money because he never did play them.

In the end, Al Rock was investigated by the Federal Election Commission, but he died before the case was closed. I wonder how our world might have changed if my mother had served in Congress. I wonder how my mother would have lived her life and how she would have remembered it. One thing I do know is that my mother has no regrets. In Susie's world, life happens and *"there it is."*

སྲ

Later in the day, I call Hilary Cleveland to tell her about Susie's Alzheimer's. She is surprised.

"The last time I saw your mother, she was her usual airy self." she says. Then Hilary begins reminiscing about the 1980 campaign, when she campaigned for my mother while her husband supported Judd Gregg. Hilary is a classy and courageous woman who has always been a loyal friend to my mother.

"Remember when your aunt Sally rode in the Fourth of July parades, pretending that she was Susan, so that you could cover twice as many parades?" Hilary asks. "Every woman candidate needs a wife. Susan had her twin sister!"

Hilary knows all about candidates' wives. For twenty years, she held down the fort in New Hampshire, raising a large family while her husband served in Congress in Washington. Hilary realizes more than most friends just how much our lives would have changed if my mother had won the election. Wife, mother, candidate, and congresswoman—now there's a juggling act!

CHAPTER FIFTEEN

PARADISE POINT

FRIDAY AFTERNOON, Brad and I take the boys to the mall in search of long pants. Zach has grown a foot in a year and a half and Travis is not far behind. I can still remember my brother Alan complaining that his pants were always too short. Now I realize why. Growing teenage boys need new pants every other month.

After an hour of "malling," I have had enough. My mind keeps wandering back to the conversation with my mother about coming to terms with the end of her life. I leave Brad and the boys to go up to Newfound Lake for dinner with my parents.

This weekend is our "McLane Thanksgiving," now celebrated over Columbus Day weekend at the lake. Cousins from around New England will gather to celebrate our family traditions, wearing Scottish kilts, singing, and eating turkey and plenty of pie.

In eighty years, our traditions have evolved from a formal dinner with the Episcopal bishop and square dancing at my grandmother's house in Manchester, to everyone bringing the vegetables and pies and singing around the fire at Newfound Lake.

Over the years, Susie has become the most McLane of all, wearing the Scottish tartan with pride and welcoming the family with open arms. In June 2001, we entertained more than a hundred relatives for a four-day McLane reunion. We hired a caterer for the first time. This weekend, we are only half the clan and Susie plans to cook two enormous turkeys.

I arrive Friday evening to a peaceful scene of my parents relaxing in rocking chairs on the porch and watching the sun set over the lake. The foliage is reaching peak colors, with brilliant reds and glowing yellows reflecting on the deep blue water.

Sparkling orange leaves drift from the trees overhead, floating down to land on the dark water. The hillside across the lake is a tapestry of colors, deep greens mixed with bright patches of crimson and gold. The view is breathtaking as the sun sinks behind the hills and the clouds take on a rosy glow.

My parents are surprised by my early arrival. They have been reading aloud the early chapters of Susie's story. I am relieved that both my mother and my father are pleased, and willing to share their past, including a few family secrets.

We talk and laugh about the memories as my parents begin opening their hearts and minds about the changes in their lives. Capturing my mother's story is becoming a catalyst for more candid family conversations.

We are intrigued about the way memories are made and kept over the years. I share Shenk's theory that "the act of remembering itself generates new memories":

Overlap, in other words, is not only built into the biology of memory. It is the very basis of memory – and identity. New memory traces are laid down on top of a foundation of old memories, and old memories can only be recalled in a context of recent experiences. Imagine a single painting being created over the course of a lifetime on one giant canvas. Every brush stroke coming into contact with many others can be seen only in the context of those prior strokes – and also instantly alters those older strokes. Because of this, no recorded experience can ever be fully distinct from anything else. Whether one likes it or not, the past is always informed by the present, and vice versa.

As we talk about our memories of events in our lives, we begin to realize that each of us has a different perspective, based on our age and stage at the time and our role in the family. Added to the challenge of writing the story of my mother's life is the reality that her own recollections are clouded by the "plaques and tangles" of Alzheimer's spreading through her brain. Shenk describes the progression of the disease as we are living it right now:

The middle stages bring the end of ambiguity. The subtle cues that something was not quite right – so easy to miss a few years ago – are now bright, self-reflecting signposts of decline, impossible to avoid. Conversation is now pockmarked with lost names and empty recollections. Times and dates have become fungible. Concentration wanes. The mind is now clearly ebbing.

My sister Robin arrives as we sit down for dinner in front of the fire. The four of us have a delightful evening, sharing stories from our family life decades ago. Robin is the oldest and I am the youngest of the five children. Eight years apart, our memories are often different, even of the same experiences.

Certain themes in our childhood transcend these differences, however, such as our mother's passion for nature and for cooking. We laugh as we recall gathering wild grapes for grape jelly, picking apples for applesauce in the fall, and collecting sap from the trees for maple syrup in the spring.

Robin remembers our pet goat, Brigadoon, who died from eating varnish off the picnic table. We all remember our dog, Highland Fling, but everyone is surprised to hear me say that he was eventually put to sleep when he bit the neighbor's child (who pulled his tail and ears.) Robin was away at college by then and my parents were busy with their lives, but I'll never forget how guilty I felt for letting the dog out without a leash.

The conversation turns to our manuscript and Susie's candor about her pregnancy and marriage during her freshman year in college. Talking with Robin openly for the first time, my parents' tone is lighthearted and loving, as if they are relieved to finally tell her about her birth.

My parents relate the story of their engagement and how happy they were to marry and move to England, where Robin was born.

"We took a pound off your birth weight when we cabled home to our parents so that they would think you were premature," my father says with a smile. Then he reflects, "There were three big decisions that I made in my life without consulting my parents: enlisting in the Air Force, marrying Susan, and not practicing law with Dad. My parents never laid down the law, but there was a powerful pull to follow their direction."

The theme of open communication inspires us all weekend. On Saturday afternoon, Robin and I go for a walk with her dog on the Audubon trails along the lake at Paradise Point. After graduating from Harvard in 1971, Robin taught junior high school in Concord. Then she moved to Portsmouth, married political activist Robin Read, and served in the legislature when their daughter Marion was born in 1982. While raising Marion, my sister coordinated curriculum for the College for Lifelong Learning. Now she is working on her Ph.D. at the University of

New Hampshire. As we walk through the colorful woods, we talk about our parents and how they are coping with aging and Alzheimer's disease.

I recount to Robin my conversation with Malcolm over breakfast this morning about the options in their lives as the illness progresses. For the first time, he has expressed an interest in someone coming to the house in the morning to be with Susie while he goes to the office. Right now, she revels in her domesticity, cooking and doing laundry every day. But he realizes that some day, perhaps soon, she will need help around the house.

He also recognizes now that she may decline to an advanced stage before they can move into Kendal several years from now. I tell Robin about his idea that Susie could move to The Birches in Concord for full-time care while he stays in their condo and visits her every day.

Robin and I are relieved, both by our father's planning and by his open and honest approach to their future. Considering his denial less than a year ago, he has come a long way. We talk about how we can support our father and help him cope in the months ahead.

When we return from our walk, Susie is presiding over the Thanksgiving meal preparations. Everyone is in awe of her cooking, roasting two twenty-five pound turkeys all day and making the gravy before the dinner is served.

Cousins begin arriving, wearing their red and green McLane plaid kilts and carrying mashed potatoes, squash, cider, and pies, lots of pies. In the end, we have fifty-four children and adults for dinner and more than a dozen pies, a fair ratio by any standard.

My sister Debbie's family arrives in several different cars, Ashley driving from Williams, then Maile and Laurel from Milton Academy. There are hugs and kisses all around each time someone walks in the door, followed by conversation and laughter as cousins connect once again. Debbie and Peter arrive late from the wedding of an old friend in Vermont, the grandson of our grandfather's law partner. New England is a small world.

Debbie is a teacher who became the quintessential stay-at-home mom when her girls were young. After graduating from Harvard, she married her ski team coach, Peter Carter, who practices law in Norwich, Vermont. While raising their three girls, she volunteered in the schools and served on the school board for years. When her oldest daughter went off to college, Debbie went back to Harvard for her master's degree. She will turn fifty in January, with plenty of time in her life to become a school principal.

The evening is a jolly affair, with children of all ages running through the house playing sardines, while the adults sip sherry and talk on the porch and by the fire. Pasquaney, our ancestral home on the lake, was a twenty-fifth-wedding-anniversary present in 1909 from my great-grandfather Charles Parker Bancroft to his wife, Susan, known fondly as Gaga. My grandmother Elisabeth and her sister Jane brought their eight children here every summer beginning in the 1920s. My father and his siblings have decades of fond memories, of swimming and sailing on the lake and of hiking in the White Mountains.

When we were growing up in the 1950s and '60s, we would come to Pasquaney every July with dozens of cousins. My generation has our own memories of water skiing, tennis, and performing in plays, like *Peter Pan* and *The Wizard of Oz*. As we trade stories and memories, it becomes clear that everyone has a different perspective on the same experience of summers on Newfound Lake.

We begin to realize that events in the early 1960s changed life at Pasquaney. My older cousins' memories of my grandparents presiding over Sunday dinner on the lawn with the whole family are very different from the younger cousins' recollections of life after my grandfather's stroke. Robin is surprised to learn that half of the family never even heard my grandfather speak. My sister talks about our grandfather's passion for nature and his hobby of banding birds.

The Thanksgiving dinner is quite spectacular, turkey with all the fixings, vegetables from various gardens, and endless pies for dessert. When everyone is satiated from the meal and conversation, we clear out the living room for the oldest family tradition of all, "performances." Beginning with the youngest, one by one we stand in front of the fire and share a talent, a story, or a memory with the clan.

When we were young, Susie wrote elaborate songs for us to sing. We all practiced our musical instruments in preparation for the big moment. Then, in the early 1960s, my brother Alan made a momentous decision for a young boy in a family filled with high expectations. When his turn came, Alan simply said in a small voice, "I pass."

With those two words, Alan became the most powerful person I knew as a child. This ten-year-old boy with red hair and freckles turned the tide of family history. He empowered an entire generation to defy authority. Alan has marched to his own drum ever since. To this day, we are grateful for his perspective on family expectations.

So now the experience is entirely voluntary. The youngest cousins love to perform. Tonight's talents are especially impressive. Mira is wearing a miniature McLane kilt with a black velvet jacket and white Peter Pan collar. She performs a play with finger puppets about a princess finding her prince.

Nicholas teaches us the alphabet in sign language. Emily performs a Scottish sword dance. Tucker plays the clarinet and Alec exhibits his drawings of skateboarders. The talent begins to peter out by the teenagers, so I decide to read the early chapters of Susie's story to my extended family.

As I read, I look up from time to time at the faces of the people I love. My mother seems proud and pleased. My father smiles through his tears. My siblings and cousins listen with open faces, as my nieces begin to cry. By the end, everyone is wiping away tears.

I realize that my parents and I are farther along in this journey. Each person in the room has different memories of Susie, depending on age and stage in life and role in the family. Each one will come to terms with her decline in his or her own way. Each person's perception is her own reality. None of us can do anything about my mother aging, except to be here with her, living in the moment, appreciating what life has to offer. This is the life lesson we are learning from Susie as she slips away.

We sing traditional Scottish songs and old family favorites late into the night. On Sunday morning, we gather around the kitchen table for breakfast, with Susie's homemade applesauce, English muffins, and coffee. We discuss our reactions to the events of September 11 and compare how our lives have changed. We feel the urgency of our time together. We each renew our commitment to family gatherings and traditions that once seemed confining but now feel comforting.

My brother Alan is quiet when the kitchen is crowded with talkative McLanes, but later he and I drink another cup of coffee and talk about his life. Alan built his own house on the side of a mountain in Jackson with a view of Mount Washington. When his girls were young, their house had no electricity and was accessible only by snowmobile all winter long. When Laura and Carrie became teenagers, Alan and Alice moved the family down the hill to a house with running water and electricity in the winter.

Years ago, Alan handled the horses for the sleigh rides in Jackson. Now he is working on his apprenticeship to become a master electrician. Today as we talk, I realize that I am listening more carefully and giving him more time to respond. Learning from my time with Susie, I let Alan finish his sentences without interrupting his train of thought. I learn more about his life in half an hour than I have in years of holiday visits.

Later, when Susie comes into the kitchen, I give her a big hug. "How are you feeling?" I ask.

"I'm happy," she answers. "I'm having a good time . . . but I can't talk."

"Now you know how Alan has felt in this noisy family all these years," I say, thinking about our visit this morning. "It's tough to get a word in edgewise when you are surrounded by McLanes."

"Yes," she says, then adds thoughtfully, "and like me, he didn't go to college."

I realize how it must have felt for Susie, joining the McLane family when she was only eighteen and spending the rest of her life surrounded by lawyers, Rhodes scholars, and Dartmouth professors.

My mother's remark is the first time in my life that I truly understand her transition from wife and mother to legislator and congressional candidate. The "most powerful woman in New Hampshire" is once again trying to be heard above the cacophony of our family. All we have to do is listen carefully to hear her wisdom.

CHAPTER SIXTEEN

THE SIXTH FRIDAY: MOTHER NATURE

THE ANTHRAX SCARE is the news of the day on National Public Radio as I drive to my mother's condo on Friday morning. Terror is literally in the air, arriving in an envelope addressed to Tom Brokaw at NBC News. The assistant who opened his mail developed a dark lesion on her skin that has tested positive for anthrax. The fear sinks into us, spreading up and down the East Coast with the FBI warning of another terrorist attack suspected this weekend.

My father joins us, watching from the couch, as my mother and I settle into our chairs by the fireplace. As I begin taping, my parents talk about attending an event this week for the New Hampshire Humanities Council with seven hundred people at the Center of New Hampshire. My mother exclaims,

I kissed the speaker! Malcolm, what was his name?

"Michael Beschloss, the presidential scholar."

Yes, that's it. I knew him in Washington. I couldn't say anything, so I just kissed him. He gave the perfect speech!

"Brad said that you were so courageous greeting everyone in the crowd. Several people mentioned to me this week your courage and candor, telling everyone 'I'm fine, but I have Alzheimer's.' People are surprised to hear the news, but impressed with your reaction." Susie is smiling. "Were you comfortable the whole evening?" I ask.

I was completely comfortable. I think that I have not ever gone back to what I did before. Politics was my life before. . . . I am on to a whole new era. This is a new stage in my life.

I wrote to [Governor] Jeanne Shaheen today to tell her that I can't serve any more on the Cannon Mountain Commission. I was president of the Ski Museum Board, at the bottom of the tramway at Cannon. That's why she first appointed me. . . . I told her that I have Alzheimer's and I can no longer serve.

Then I report to my mother, "Last night, Brad and I went to the Currier Gallery of Art for a fancy event. Everyone was asking about how you are doing. Burt Cohen told us about his wonderful visit with you. When I asked if you recognized him, he said 'absolutely, we were buddies in the Senate.' I told him that it was quite a compliment that you have such a strong memory of him. Burt was pleased that you remembered him so well."

Susie is delighted to hear this story about her former Senate colleague. She is pleased with her performance at a large political event.

I completely connected with Burt and with Dudley Dudley, who served with Malcolm on the Executive Council. I kissed

Walter Peterson too! He was our last, best governor, but he lost to Meldrim Thomson.

"Do you remember in 1972 when Walter Peterson lost in the Republican primary to Meldrim Thomson and the Democratic candidate was just as bad?" I watch her face carefully for any sign of recognition.

Susie listens intently as I continue: "I remember we were making applesauce in the kitchen with Alan. Daddy came home from work and announced that he was going to run for governor as an Independent. You went right to the telephone to order the bumper stickers. Then you came back and started planning the campaign, right there in the kitchen."

I remember it all! Malcolm ran for governor as an Independent. We only had eight weeks to campaign between the primary and the general election. I remember being very proud of him because he was for a broad-based tax. It was very real, incredibly real, because it was fair taxation, way back then.

We all have memories of my father's campaign for governor. "I remember driving you to Hanover to give a speech," I tell her. "I had just turned sixteen. We were halfway there when you turned to me and said, 'Wait a minute . . . you don't have a driver's license!' A friend of yours in the legislature made arrangements for me to get my license the day after my birthday so I could help with the campaign, but you were so distracted, you didn't even know."

We laugh, as I realize that this story is typical of my life as a teenager in a busy political family. I even remember driving myself to the appointment to get my license.

My mother has her own memories of my father's campaign.

Our house was full of college kids working on the campaign. Robin came home from California. Donald and Joni came home from Brown with Erik. Debbie came up on the

*weekends from Harvard. A whole group of kids who worked
on Pete McCloskey's campaign for president came back to New
Hampshire to work for Malcolm's campaign for governor.*

*We ran a television ad with a crowd of supporters all lined
up to speak into the camera and say why they were voting for
Malcolm McLane for governor.*

*Election night we had a great party at the Highway Hotel.
We made big signs to record the votes in every town as they
came in over the radio. I was so proud of Malcolm! He only
got 20 percent of the vote, but that was minor compared to the
thrill of knowing that he agreed with me about taxes.*

The phone rings and we take a short break. When we
resume, I report on a story from a friend of mine about Susie at
an Audubon meeting this week. My friend Jan's mother has
Alzheimer's, too, so she was impressed when Susie spoke up at
the meeting. "Your mother had trouble talking, but what she had
to say was the most poignant moment of our whole meeting,"
Jan told me.

Apparently, the Audubon committee was considering
whether to continue with a large capital campaign in the wake
of the terrorist attacks. Some voiced concern that the time was
not right to raise funds to renovate the nature center and create
walking trails.

Then Susie offered her opinion. "People need nature, now
more than ever before. Children and their parents need to be
together in the outdoors. We need to feel the natural beauty of
the land, the trees, the flowers and the birds. We need to feel safe
again, surrounded by nature." Jan was so impressed with my
mother's insight.

Susie is clearly delighted to hear this story.

*That's just it. The idea of students going to Washington or
New York now is gone. So going on a trip to a nature center*

is just vital. I want to create a McLane trail to connect the Audubon land in Concord to the woods and fields around St. Paul's School.

"Tell me the story of how you first began birding and enjoying nature when you were a girl growing up in Hanover," I say, curious about how my mother's love of nature first began.

Sally and I woke up at six o'clock on Saturdays. Mother said she was not going to serve breakfast until seven-thirty, so we went out into the field to watch birds.

Once we saw a huge bird . . . a pileated woodpecker in a tree. We ran down to the museum to find the college ornithologist. He was teaching a class, so he brought all the students to our yard to see the woodpecker. We were eight years old. That was the beginning of my inspiration with birds.

After that, we went out every Saturday morning with him and the bird club. I took my binoculars. Sally went with me. That was what we did together on the weekends in the fall and spring.

Birding became my lifelong hobby. When you kids were growing up, I went out every Wednesday with the Concord Bird Club. But I haven't gone at all this fall. I can't remember the names of the birds anymore. I used to know the name of every bird. I could recognize all the songs, too.

The women in the bird club were just marvelous! I sent you all off to school. Then I went birding for the morning until you came home for lunch. It was a nice way to be with friends and to be in nature. Once in a while we would take a big trip to the ocean to see the shorebirds. The women knew all the birds!

I remember my mother always had her binoculars in her purse and her telescope in her car. We would stop on the side of the road wherever we were driving to see a great blue heron in a marsh or a hawk circling in the sky.

Once on Cape Cod, when I was about ten, I joined her for a day with a famous ornithologist who lived next door to my grandmother. We rose at dawn and crisscrossed the Cape until the sun went down, sighting more than one hundred different species of shore birds, songbirds, ducks, and raptors. What a day! Susie loved every minute of it, and I loved just being with her, at peace in nature, learning about all the different kinds of birds.

Now I can't recognize all the birds anymore, but I still carry my binoculars with me all the time wherever I go. I would still recognize a pileated woodpecker, but I can't tell all the warblers apart.

"You're back to the same stage of birding that I've been my whole life," I say with a laugh. "I recognize the big birds, great blue herons and hawks circling overhead. But I never could tell all those warblers with a patch of yellow or a bit of red on their wings."

My mother's face lights up as she talks about birds and nature.

When we travel, we always go to bird sanctuaries, all over the world. We buy a bird book and learn all about the new species wherever we go.

I was the president of Audubon. (I was the president of everything I ever joined!) I raised a lot of money for the Massabesic Nature Center. But now Richard [Moore] says I can't go ask for money anymore. I'm still the chair of the fund-raising committee, but I can't speak anymore.

Richard is going to the Galápagos Islands, so I gave him my journal with pictures of all the birds. He just loved it! I kept a list of every bird we saw on the trip.

When we went down the Colorado River, the boatman had never seen all the birds along the canyons. I saw sixty-eight different kinds of birds. All he saw were the big vultures and hawks and eagles, but I kept giving him my binoculars to see the little birds on the side of the river. He was so amazed. He couldn't believe his eyes!

Appreciating nature and protecting the environment were important priorities for my mother. Susie introduced 365 bills over her quarter of a century in the New Hampshire Legislature. Most of the legislation eventually passed into law, including dozens of significant environmental protections, such as funding for land conservation; passage of the Shoreline Protection Act; and preservation of two endangered species, the Karner Blue butterfly and the Showy Ladyslipper.

As I listen to my mother talking about her love of birding, I realize that she has passed along to us her appreciation of nature. Yesterday I watched the Canada geese flying south in their V formation high in the sky. This morning I saw two dozen wild turkeys in the field at Dimond Hill Farm on my way into town.

Brad saw a coyote in the orchard on our road and I came across two black bears on my walk in the woods down by the river. Nature surrounds us, if we take the time to look. Patience is a virtue. Nature is the reward. We need to feel the natural beauty of the land to feel safe again.

As we wind up our taping, my father reflects on their life at this stage of Alzheimer's disease. "One thing that's interesting is that Susie can continue to do some things perfectly well. She can go shopping alone. She can drive anywhere when I'm in the car and around town on her own," Malcolm says.

"Susie still deals with all the mail. She has her own checkbook to write charitable contributions from her own Social Security checks. She keeps busy around the house with laundry and all. Her cooking is still terrific!

"But it all takes time," my father concludes with a sigh. "Everything takes longer than before."

Then my parents tell me about visiting Kendal yesterday for an orientation session for the folks on the waiting list. Apparently, the list is very long and moving slowly. My parents now realize that they will not be moving to Hanover for several years.

"People are living longer, especially if they live at Kendal!" Malcolm jokes. Susie chimes in,

> *It was nice to hear what other people thought about moving into Kendal. The woman doctor gave a wonderful talk about aging.* [She pauses, searching for the right words.]
>
> *But we are perfectly happy here for a while. Then I think that I want to go to The Birches, the new Alzheimer's unit in Concord, and let Malcolm stay right here at home.*

"I would love to go with you to check it out, Momma," I say, relieved that my mother has broached the subject of her future care. I share a story with her.

"My friend Jane's mother lives at The Birches. She is very happy. Jane kept her mother at home on their farm as long as she could with round-the-clock help. Her mother moved into The Birches last spring.

"When Jane brought her mother home for a visit, she said, 'Oh, what a beautiful farm. I wonder who lives here.' Jane was overcome. Her mother had lived on that farm for more than sixty years." I watch Susie's face for her reaction as I continue.

"Jane visits her mother now every day as she presides over teatime, watching out for all the residents and making sure they aren't left out. The socialization is just what her mother needed to feel better about herself." My mother is smiling now, as she says,

Ellen Sheridan is going to come back to set me up with the Alzheimer's support group. So I will do that.

We talk about how Susie has been so aware of the changes in her life and willing to talk about her decline openly. When my grandmother had Alzheimer's disease in the 1970s, nobody talked about her decline until she was too far gone to understand what was happening to her.

We are hopeful that my mother's openness can help others with Alzheimer's disease and their families to cope and to connect while they go on living their lives. Many people mention to me that their parents are beginning to slip away. I encourage them to spend time with their parents now. Live in the moment. Get past the denial. Live life together again, while you can. Savor your last dance together.

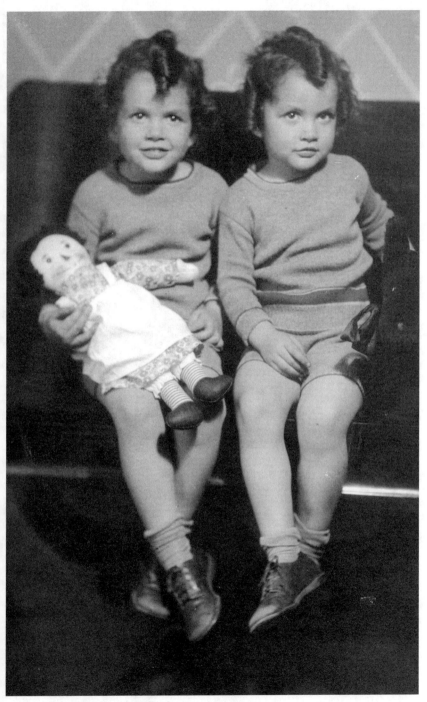

The twins, Sally and Susan Neidlinger (1932)

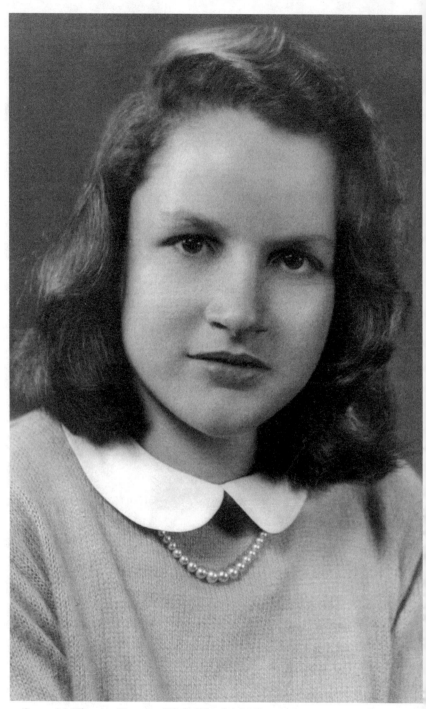

Susan Neidlinger, Hanover High School (1944)

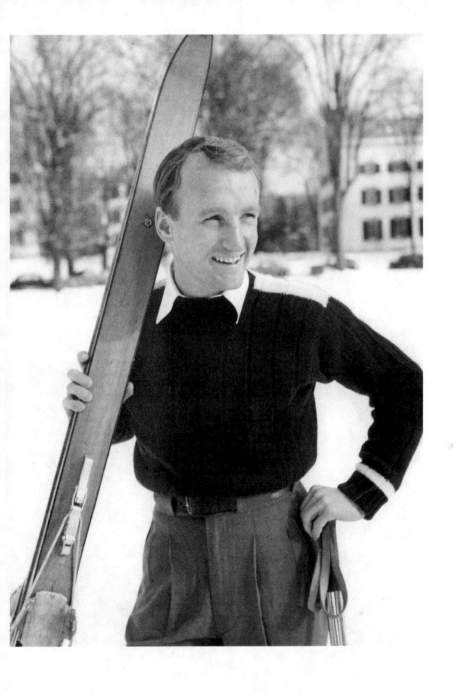

Malcolm McLane, Captain of the Dartmouth Ski Team (1948)

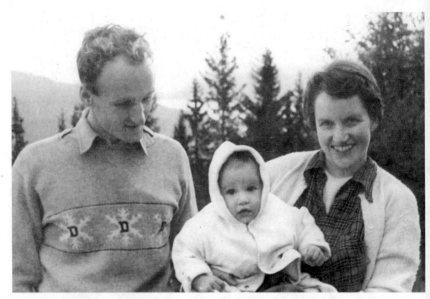

Malcolm and Susan McLane with Robin in Norway (1949)

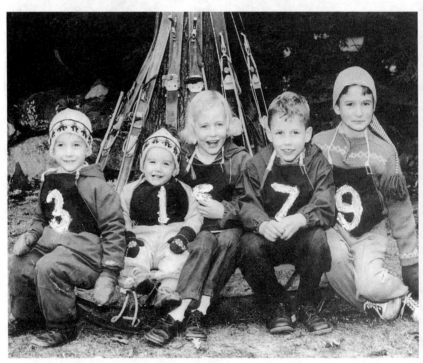

*Alan, Annie, Debbie, Donald, and Robin McLane, 1957 Christmas card
(ages 3-1-5-7-9)*

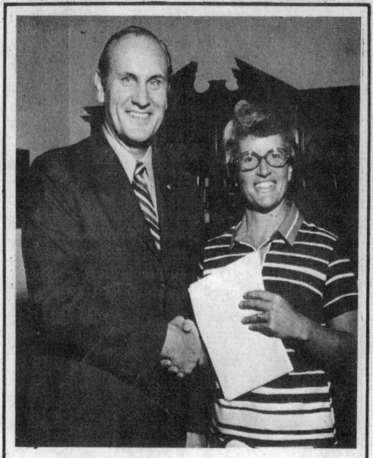

... A GOOD GOVERNOR
Deserves Good Support in the Legislature
RE-ELECT
SUE McLANE - WARD 4
Statewide Volunteers For Peterson, Chairman
Acting Clerk of House Ways & Means
signed: Susan N. McLane
Concord, N.H.

Re-elect Representative Susan McLane. Political advertisement with Governor Walter Peterson (1970)

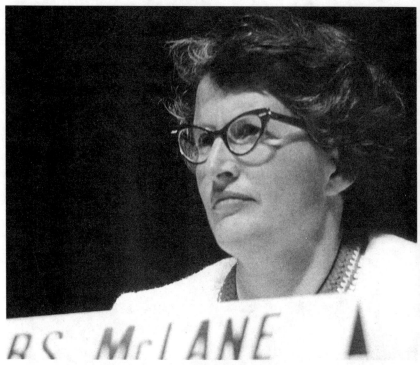

Susan McLane, World Affairs Council (1965)

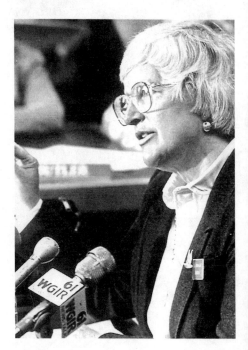

State Senator Susan McLane.
Press Conference (1988)

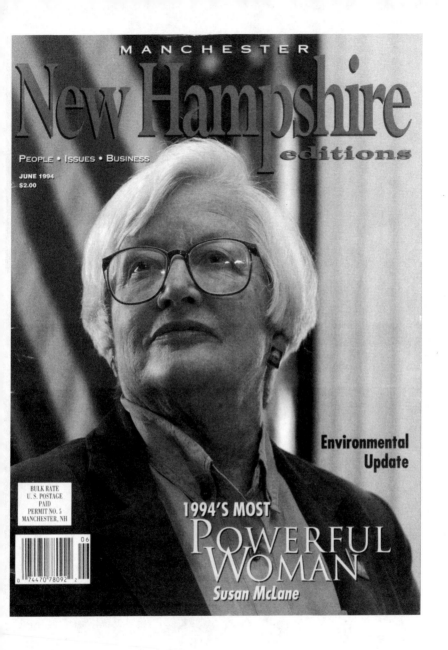

MANCHESTER

New Hampshire
editions

PEOPLE • ISSUES • BUSINESS

JUNE 1994
$2.00

Environmental
Update

BULK RATE
U. S. POSTAGE
PAID
PERMIT NO. 5
MANCHESTER, NH

1994'S MOST
POWERFUL
WOMAN
Susan McLane

Cover of New Hampshire Editions magazine (June 1994)

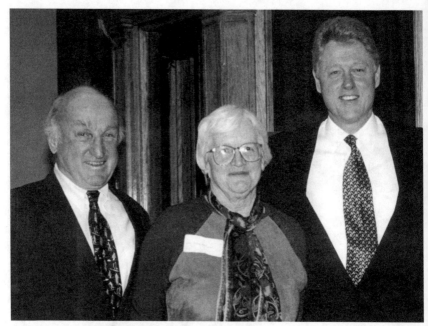

Malcolm and Susan McLane, President Bill Clinton. Capitol Center for the Arts (1996)

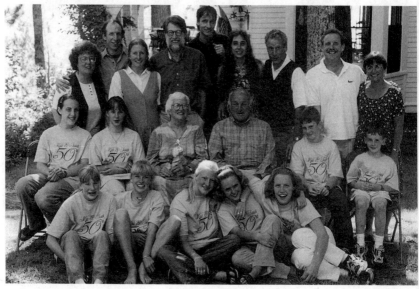

Susan and Malcolm McLane 50th Wedding Anniversary (1998). (Back row - Alice, Alan, Debbie, Peter, Eric, Lois, Donald, Brad, Annie. Middle row - Carrie, Abi, Susie, Malcolm, Zach, Travis. Front row - Laurel, Maile, Ashley, Karissa, Laura. Not pictured: Robin and Marion - travelling in India and Thailand.)

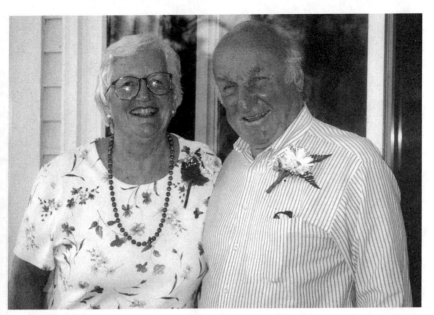

Susan and Malcolm McLane, Newfound Lake, July 2000

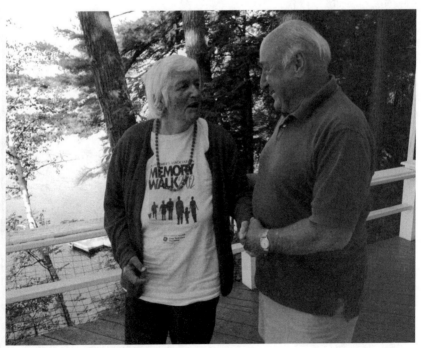

Susan and Malcolm McLane, Newfound Lake, September 2003 (photo credit: Ken Williams, Concord Monitor)

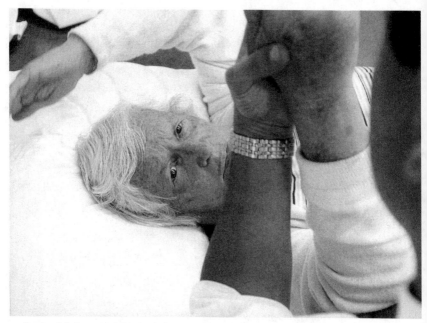

Susan McLane at physical therapy, September 2003 (photo credit: Ken Williams, Concord Monitor)

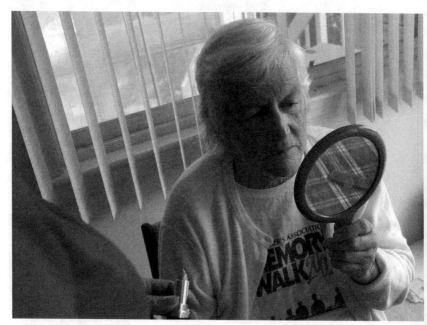

Susan McLane putting on lipstick, September 2003 (photo credit: Ken Williams, Concord Monitor)

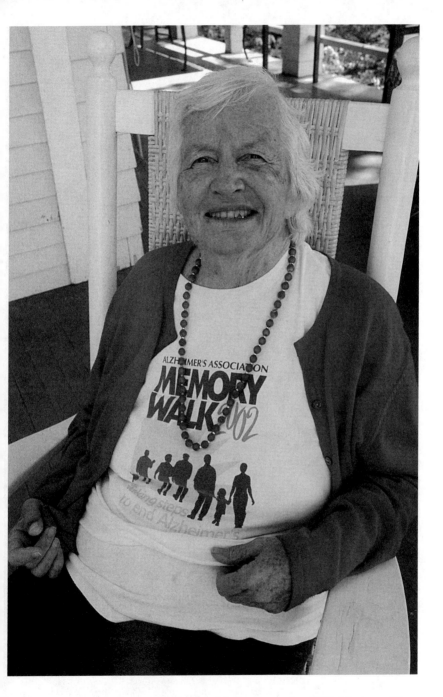

Susan McLane on the porch, Newfound Lake, September 2003 (photo credit: Ken Williams, Concord Monitor)

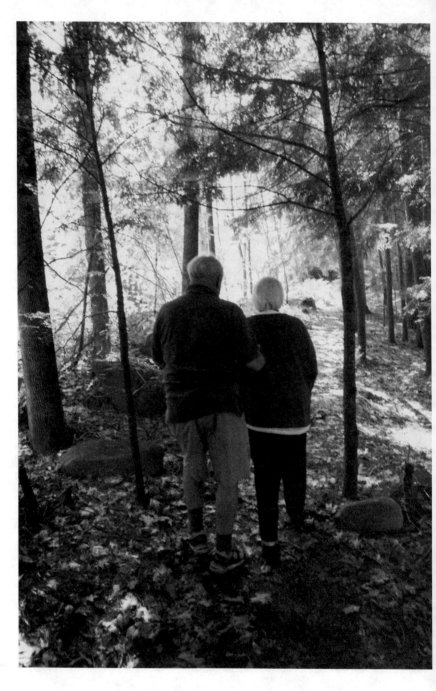

Susan and Malcolm McLane, Newfound Lake, September 2003 (photo credit: Ken Williams, Concord Monitor)

CHAPTER SEVENTEEN

HEART AND SOUL

THE QUESTIONS ARE intertwined in my mind like strands of DNA. What is a "normal" life after September 11 or after Alzheimer's disease? Uncertainty and fear weave in and out of our lives, yet we are more appreciative of every day. We are living life in the present, aware of each moment. We cherish the "small stuff," reveling in natural beauty and human kindness throughout every day.

At breakfast, the boys and I are awestruck by the sunrise over the hills, bright pink and gold reflecting off the wispy clouds. The foliage is now reaching peak colors. Brilliant red, orange, and yellow trees contrast with dark evergreens, blanketing the hills and valleys in every direction. Driving into town, my eyes seek out the most spectacular tree, then the next, and the next. We are surrounded by natural beauty. We are blessed by this season in our lives.

All day long, I appreciate the random acts of kindness of colleagues, clients, and "folks I haven't met yet" along the way. We stop to chat more often. We stay longer, talking over a cup of coffee about the news of the day or our children's latest fears. Patience is a virtue. Meaningful connection is the reward.

At a concert in remembrance of September 11, our friend Peggo Hodes sings a beautiful solo of "The Rose," a song made popular by Bette Midler. The words grip my heart, as the uncertainty of our future grips my life.

> *Some say love, it is a hunger,*
> *an endless aching need.*
> *I say love, it is a flower,*
> *and you, its only seed.*
> *It's the heart, afraid of breaking,*
> *that never learns to dance.*
> *It's the dream, afraid of waking,*
> *that never takes the chance.*
> *It's the one who won't be taken*
> *who cannot seem to give,*
> *And the soul afraid of dyin',*
> *that never learns to live.*

I am reminded once again of my mother, who has learned to live by not being afraid to die.

ॐ

Humor slowly slips back into our lives. A friend sends an e-mail message urging the United States not to invade Afghanistan, but instead to round up all the women living under the Taliban and send them to college. Another message suggests that the CIA capture Osama bin Laden, give him a sex change, and send him back to live as a woman under his own regime.

Alzheimer's disease, we discover, has its own offbeat humor. Malcolm chuckles whenever Susie says to one of her own children over the phone, "You'll have to speak with my husband about that."

On Saturday night, over dinner with friends, we laugh together as Lucia and I exchange stories about our mothers. Lucia's mother suffered a brain aneurysm that catapulted her overnight from early Alzheimer's to a much later stage. Living in a nursing home in Maine now, Lucia's mother can no longer perform simple daily tasks, like getting dressed, preparing meals, and using a telephone. She is completely lost in time and space, never knowing the time of day, the day of the week, or even the season.

One story stands out as a turning point in Lucia's learning to appreciate what was left of her wonderful and wise mother. She brought her mother along on a trip with her son Sam to Plimoth Plantation, thinking that she would enjoy the site, the gardens, and the history. Sam and Lucia had fun talking to the interpreters dressed in costume and role-playing characters from the Seventeenth century. They asked lots of questions about life on the plantation, why they left England, and about the hardships of the first winter in the New World. Lucia's mother listened attentively.

Later Lucia asked her mother if she enjoyed the visit to Plimoth. "It was terrible," her mother replied. "I felt so sorry for those poor people living in such dark and dingy houses. I don't understand why they would ever leave England to live like that."

Lucia realized that no amount of explaining could help her mother understand that the "Pilgrims" were only actors. She no longer had any concept of time. Four centuries ago was indistinguishable from the present. So Lucia bit her tongue and agreed with her mother that the houses were dark. She, too, hoped that life would improve for those poor women. Lucia focused on her mother's compassion. She told her mother how much she admired her for always caring about people less fortunate.

When Lucia finishes her story, we chuckle over the actors going home to cook dinner in a microwave oven and watch television. Alzheimer's disease is serious and sobering, but we realize that humor is essential in our lives now.

❧

On a peaceful walk along the river on Sunday morning, my friend Susan, an infectious disease doctor at Concord Hospital, is worrying about antibiotic supplies and disaster protocols. She has been called to an emergency meeting with state officials about anthrax and bioterrorism. The threat feels closer to home now.

In Susie's world, the enemy comes from within. Plaques and tangles are invading her brain. Freedom of thought and of speech are threatened. My mother's life is changing week to week, day by day.

On Sunday afternoon, Lucia comes over for tea to talk about my Fridays with Susie. Lucia is my mentor, recounting stories about her mother and guiding me through the stages and moods of Alzheimer's disease. In turn, I am her interpreter, giving her new perspective on the whole experience.

Lucia wonders if my mother's candid and open approach to Alzheimer's could ultimately change the course of her disease. As we open our hearts and minds to the reality of Alzheimer's disease, we begin to find new meaning in life and in love.

I find myself softly singing "The Rose."

> *It's the heart, afraid of breaking,*
> *that never learns to dance.*
> *It's the dream, afraid of waking,*
> *that never takes the chance.*

It's the one who won't be taken
who cannot seem to give.
And the soul afraid of dyin',
that never learns to live.

As the autumn leaves fall off the trees, the bright red partridge berries peek through their shiny green leaves. Every fall, as the natural world around us fades into winter, Susie picks the berries and greens to make wreaths for Christmas.

All winter long, as the wind blows and the snow blankets the forest, her partridge berry wreath is a beacon of natural beauty and hope in my mother's life. Nestled in a silver bowl and nurtured every day, the wreath is a symbol of her heart and soul. Autumn is the season to pick partridge berries, and to hold hope close to our hearts. Autumn is the season of our last dance, a time to hold love close to our soul.

CHAPTER EIGHTEEN

WISHFUL THINKING

DURING THE WEEK, my colleague Lucy calls with urgency in her voice.

"Annie, are you okay.?" she asks.

"Sure, I'm fine. Why?" I wonder.

"Well, your mother . . . are you okay with what's happening with your mother? I mean, I know this must be so hard for you, but I'm just wondering. Are you okay?" Lucy sounds very worried.

"Yes, it's difficult for all of us. But I'm fine. I appreciate you asking, but we're okay. My mother and I are both enjoying our time together on Fridays and my father is becoming a saint," I reassure her.

"But, you're not running for governor, are you?" she asks, sounding shocked and surprised.

"What? No, I'm not running for governor. Whatever made you think that?" Now I'm confused, too.

"Well, I just spoke with a client who saw your mother last week at the Humanities Council dinner. Apparently, she told him that you are running for governor. Then she told him how much money you make!" Lucy is laughing now.

"Oh my God!" I am laughing, too, but I am mortified. "Maybe we're not okay. Thanks for telling me anyway," I say, laughing with tears in my eyes.

Once again in Susie's world our public and private lives merge, with a few new twists and turns. I suddenly think of the T.V. cameraman on the State House lawn on September 11, who said to me, "The world will never be the same again." Our life is changing again, in subtle and mysterious ways. The question now is how to live life amid the changes. The question is how to reconcile my mother's wishful thinking about me with my wishful thinking about her.

CHAPTER NINETEEN

THE SEVENTH FRIDAY: 'EVERYBODY'S ALL AMERICAN'

ON FRIDAY MORNING, my mother comes to my house for our taping, so that I can drive to Hanover afterward to meet my old Dartmouth Ski Team friends for lunch. Susie is wearing Sally's red cashmere sweater. She looks radiant, smiling with a twinkle in her eye.

My mother enjoys our Friday visits. She looks forward to talking about her life, then and now. Although she repeats some stories and often wanders off track, I am still impressed by the details of her memory from years ago. She begins today at the beginning again, then moves on to a new story.

I am just so appreciative of you and Malcolm. It's funny about Malcolm. He always thought that he was superior to me. I married him when I was eighteen. Although I was the freshman class president, I really enjoyed the babies. I had my first baby in England, my second baby in Cambridge, my third and fourth babies in Hanover, and then my fifth baby in Concord.

I had no medicine when Robin was born. I had her in an hour and a half, delivered by a nineteen-year-old midwife. In England, they wanted me to nurse the baby. But when Donald was born, I had to say I wanted to nurse him, instead of the other way around. I nursed all five of my babies. [She smiles proudly.]

Malcolm was never allowed to attend the births. When you were born, nobody even told him. He went home from the waiting room around midnight. I was knocked out cold for the birth. During the night, the cleaning lady told me that I had a baby boy! But in the morning, they brought you to my room. That's when Malcolm and I learned we had another girl.

I remember how hard my mother tried to witness the birth of a grandchild. She helped right through Robin's labor, but missed Marion's birth by minutes when she gave Malcolm a ride home from the hospital late at night. She and Brad were my coaches when I was in labor with Zach, but he was born by surprise cesarean in the middle of the night. Finally, when my son Travis, the last grandchild, was born, my mother watched the miracle of birth for the first time.

Susie loves hearing these stories now, but she cannot remember any of the details. Whole chapters of her memory have slipped away. But she continues to find meaning in her life.

We have had a very pleasant week. The reason is that Malcolm doesn't go to work more than an hour or two in the morning. Then we have the whole day together!

We drove up to Cannon Mountain and through the Notch to Jackson. We took Alan out to dinner. Then we spent the

night at the house. It was just Alan for dinner. That was so much better talking with him alone. He talked all about becoming an electrician.
[Susie stops talking and I realize that she is staring at the pictures of my family on the mantel.]
These pictures are so beautiful that I can't believe it! They are just marvelous!

I try focusing our time this week on my mother's parents and her life growing up in Hanover. Although my original idea was to capture the story of my mother's political career, her memory is strongest the farther back in her life we explore. Following her lead, I decide to go with the flow. Life is too short now, and too long before, to care about chronology any longer.

My father, "Pudge" Neidlinger, was the Dean of Dartmouth, so he was out of the picture much of the time. I never got to know him very well. He painted pictures when he wasn't working, so we didn't see him very much.
[She points out several of my grandfather's paintings in my house, including the Main Street on Nantucket and Dartmouth Hall.]
I loved my mother completely! When she died, I went to her best friend to tell her and she said, "Thank goodness. The lucky duck!"

I will never forget the scene myself. My parents and I were visiting my grandmother Marion, known lovingly as Grammy, at her home in Chatham on Cape Cod over Labor Day weekend in 1979. My grandfather had died in the spring of 1978, just before I graduated from Dartmouth.

Grammy was going blind and was sad to be living alone. A graduate of Sweet Briar, my grandmother had devoted her entire life to raising a family and taking care of my grandfather. Her only pleasure now was listening to talking books and reminiscing with friends.

One morning during our visit, my mother was resting with the flu upstairs while my father was reading in the living room. I was taking a bath when my grandmother burst into the bathroom.

"I'm so sorry, Ann, but I think I'm going to lose my lunch," she said, rushing to the toilet. Grammy was flustered to intrude upon my bath. I knew right away that she was not feeling well.

I dressed quickly, then settled my grandmother into her bed, thinking she had the flu. Her last words to me were, "Ann, I hope you can manage making your own breakfast."

"Grammy, I'm twenty-three years old. I think I can fix my own breakfast." I replied with a laugh.

Over the next half hour, I kept checking on my grandmother from the doorway, so as not to disturb her rest. She was sleeping peacefully each time I checked, but eventually I realized that she had not moved in a long time. I went closer to check on her. Only then did I realize that my grandmother had died in her sleep of a heart attack, quietly, without sound or struggle.

Grammy's best friend was jealous that her final moments were peaceful, sleeping in her own bed with her family around. I remember my grandmother's doctor telling us that he wished more families could experience death this way. When I expressed regret that I hadn't called an ambulance, the doctor told me that my grandmother would have died on the highway, rushing to the hospital with sirens blaring. Her doctor was certain that Grammy would prefer falling asleep peacefully, in her own bed, wearing her sneakers.

"Tell me about your life growing up with your mother," I ask, hoping to learn more about my mother's relationship with her own mother.

Every summer we took the train and the ferry to Nantucket. My sisters and I spent the summer with my mother in a little cottage out at Surfside next to the Coast Guard station. We lived next door to a Dartmouth professor who grew up on Nantucket, with his three boys (I can't remember his name).

We slept late, until eight o'clock. Then we got up and had breakfast. It was ten o'clock by then, when we went to the beach. We went birding in the afternoon on our bicycles. I just remember it as so blissful. We never had a bad word!

Pudge came for two weeks, so we were on our own with Mother the rest of the time. He would paint along the beach, hunched over his easel. He was six feet four inches tall, an all-American college football player and Dean of Dartmouth College. [she pauses] *That was just it.*

When we were growing up, Pudge was legendary for kicking a fifty-one-yard field goal for Dartmouth against Harvard in 1922. My classmate Nick Lowery kicked a fifty-one-yard field goal in 1976, before going on to a distinguished NFL career. Watching from the stands at the Harvard-Dartmouth game in Cambridge, Pudge was pleased that Nick tied his record but didn't surpass it.

Once when the twins were young, Susan and Sally convinced their father to demonstrate his athletic prowess to a skeptical student. According to legend, Dean Neidlinger put on his fedora, walked the skeptic down to the football field, and had him hold the ball on the forty-one-yard line (the goal posts were ten yards behind the end zone then). Pudge repeated the kick in his tweed suit and street shoes, without ever removing his hat. Then he turned around and kicked another fifty-one-yard field goal in the opposite direction, for good measure.

I'm curious about whether my grandfather's athletic achievements influenced his daughters when they were growing up.

> *Daddy drove Sally and me to all our ski races on the weekends because we couldn't drive until we were sixteen. We skied at Moosilauke and Cannon before there were any ski lifts. We hiked up the trail and learned the race course on the way up. It was better that way. We knew the trail when we raced down.*

> *Once I stopped to talk to a friend who was hiking up while I was skiing down. My father was not impressed! Sally and I would win, unless we were beaten by the Wurtle twins, from Canada. I remember those years as sensational! I was very happy.*

"What did Pudge and Grammy think when you and Daddy were married?" I ask, curious about her parents' reaction.

> *Well, I was president of my class at Mount Holyoke. I roomed with a gal from the South in the front of the dormitory on the first floor. I told my parents that I was pregnant. They were sympathetic from then on. I told them that Malcolm was not willing to go to Oxford without me.*

> *I was completely unaware of their reaction, because I was so aware of my reaction. Whatever they thought wasn't going to faze me in the slightest.*

> *We were married in the church in Lenox, near Mount Holyoke. Our parents all came to the wedding. My sister Mary was my maid of honor and Malcolm's brother John was the best man. I walked down the aisle with my father and the minister performed the ceremony.*

> *After the service, we went to the minister's house for a reception. It was the thirtieth of April, but it was snowing*

when we left. Everyone threw snowballs at us as we got into the car!

"What? You had a church wedding?" I ask in amazement. "We never knew that. There's not a single photograph."

I am astonished. My mother put on three wonderful weddings for my sisters and me at Newfound Lake, but I have never even heard the story of her wedding. The only picture I ever saw is one of my mother wearing a suit, ducking into a car. All these years, I assumed that my parents were married in a ceremony in the office of a justice of the peace, then whisked away in secrecy. Little did I realize, they were ducking into the car to escape snowballs.

No, there's not a single photograph . . . [She pauses.] Anyway, I was in love with him. So I was very flattered about marrying him. . . . It was completely unrelated to the pregnancy. [She smiles.]

"I think that's a wonderful story," I say. "That's the whole point." I am utterly amazed that we never knew this story, but I am pleased to hear my mother tell it now. She is opening her heart and her world for us to share.

We went to the Catskills for our honeymoon, but I had only one night free from Mount Holyoke. So we came back Sunday night and stayed at the College Inn.

"Did you finish school that semester?" I ask.

Yes. I took an exam in the morning and got married in the afternoon. I took the rest of my exams early. . . . I went back to my fiftieth reunion at Mount Holyoke last June.

After my exams were over, I went back to Hanover to be with Malcolm. We went to Newfound Lake for the rest of our honeymoon. That summer, we worked together on Sel Hannah's farm in Franconia.

Then we went to England. Malcolm was a Rhodes scholar studying at Oxford. Robin was born right before Christmas. The next summer when Robin was a baby, my parents came to visit with Sally, because they couldn't leave her home alone.[She laughs.]

We traveled around Europe, five of us and the baby. Malcolm drove and Pudge sat in front in the little car. Sally and I sat with Mother in the back. Robin was in the "carry-cot" on our knees! When we stopped to eat in a restaurant, Malcolm would ask the chef to heat up Robin's bottle in the kitchen. . . . I was so close to Malcolm by then that I felt distant from Sally.

Sally went to college in Colorado. Then she married John and moved to California. She had three babies, all boys. The most marvelous thing I ever did was to go out for two and a half months to be with her before she died.

Mary was the oldest. She graduated from Mount Holyoke. Then she married Bob and they lived in Cohasset. She had three babies, too, two boys and a girl.

I remember the summer of 1961, when we all vacationed together in Brewster on Cape Cod. The three families shared a house overlooking the ocean. Pudge and Grammy rented a little cottage next door. The children would gather around Pudge while he was painting the beach scene. I still remember my cousin Jake, age three at the time, wearing jeans and carrying a corncob pipe.

Every day we would swim from the beach at high tide. Then we would walk farther and farther out on the mudflats when the tide was low, looking for shells and sea creatures. One day, the tide came in faster than we realized. The cousins had to run across the mudflats, then finally swim with our shirts held high overhead. Jim and Jake were worried that their mother would be upset when their shorts got wet. But the older cousins knew that the adventure was well worth the risk.

My mother appreciates hearing these stories again. She doesn't remember the details, but she enjoys the feelings of fondness for her family. Then she talks about her parents when Pudge left Dartmouth in 1952 after serving as Dean of the College for twenty years.

> *When Pudge and Grammy left Dartmouth, they moved to Scarsdale. Daddy worked in New York City. We used to visit their apartment when you kids were little.*
>
> *That was so wonderful . . . because it was them, at home. We visited more often. We spent more time with Pudge and Grammy when they lived in Chatham.*
>
> *When Pudge died in the hospital in Hyannis, I didn't realize that he was going to die. Grammy had to make a decision about another surgery or letting him die. She didn't know what to do. She was so sad to let him go after all their years together.*
>
> *After Pudge died, I put in the bill for the Living Will and it passed. I worked with the lawyer for the Catholic Church. That was one of my proudest moments.*

After my grandfather died, my mother introduced the Living Will legislation in New Hampshire. She wanted other families to know the wishes of their loved ones who were dying. Susie didn't want anyone else to feel the pain Grammy had experienced, not knowing what Pudge wanted to happen at the end of his life. My mother organized a broad coalition of health care and religious groups to support the Living Will legislation. Ultimately, she even garnered the support of the Catholic Church.

The lawyer for the Catholic Diocese recently told me the story of how my mother hammered out the compromise language. Then she took him with her to Legislative Services to draft the bill. She told them, "Here's the Living Will bill and here's the language that we want. That's the way you will write it." The lawyer was so impressed with her resolve and determination. As a legislator, Susie knew how to get the job done.

After both her parents died within a year, my mother sponsored legislation to license hospice services in New Hampshire. She worked with an activist in Concord who was creating the first hospice house to provide compassionate care to dying patients. My mother became an advocate for a more humane approach to death and dying that would allow physicians to administer pain medications but withhold extraordinary measures to prolong life. Patients and families could spend their last days together living life rather than fighting death.

Now my mother's activist life is nearing an end. Like the line in "The Rose," Susie has learned how to live by not being afraid of dying. Susie explains:

> *I feel completely now that I am ready to die.*
> *It's not that I want to die, but that I am willing to die.*
> *A friend came for lunch recently who was upset about our plans to go to Egypt for a boat trip down the Nile in January. Malcolm told her not to worry about us.*
> *I just feel that I am totally into going to visit Egypt, even if it is dangerous. When we travel on the boat for ten days, I will be very relaxed. If Malcolm has paid his money and we aren't going anywhere else, why not go to Egypt?*

Talking with your parents about death and dying is like talking with your teenagers about sex. You don't want to have the conversation too soon, but you definitely don't want to have the conversation too late. I realize that I need to talk with my mother now about her wishes upon her death before she can't remember anything at all.

CHAPTER TWENTY

THE EIGHTH FRIDAY: 'NO PLACE TO HIDE'

THE FEAR OF ANTHRAX spreads from Washington and New York west to Middle America this week via the U.S. Postal Service. No one is immune from the scare. What began as a threat to our media empires and political symbols soon becomes a fact of life for ordinary Americans. Postal workers, doctors and nurses, even secretaries opening mail now work on the front line as terror slowly circles the globe.

My assistant and I talk about wearing gloves to open mail from New York and Washington. Suzanne has been cautious for several weeks, checking envelopes with care. Political leaders urge all Americans to carry on with their lives, but fear of the unknown is with us every day now.

My parents enjoyed their trip to Washington, despite the anthrax scare. Their visit with Justice Souter was thwarted by the U.S. Supreme Court closure on Friday, but they thoroughly enjoyed touring the Georgetown campus with Marion. On the weekend, they visited new friends from the Alaska trip on the eastern shore of Maryland. "The trip was perfect!" Susie exclaimed upon their return.

The leaves are falling off the trees. The nights are colder. The days are wet and gray. Halloween night is dark and drizzly. Travis and a friend defy the weather, trick-or-treating through the neighborhood as "the Scream" and an authentic John Lennon with granny glasses and a peace medallion.

I wander along behind, thinking about children in Afghanistan spooked by bombs and food falling from the sky. The packages contain Pop Tarts, along with rice and lentils, as though we are confused about our message of peace in a foreign war-torn land.

⤳

On Friday morning, my parents come to Hopkinton for a walk along the Contoocook River. The day is warm for early November. A few bronze leaves cling to the trees. The path is a carpet of crimson and gold. As we walk along the river, Susie smiles as she repeats again and again, "This is so beautiful!"

My mother is delighted with another day surrounded by natural beauty. She is charmed by the hole of a woodpecker and the sight of partridge berries buried beneath the leaves. Malcolm bends over slowly to pick the shiny green leaves and bright red berries. Susie and I crouch down to pick in our own patch a few feet away.

"Susie, do you remember how to make the wreaths?" Malcolm wonders aloud.

"I will once I start!" Susie says with confidence. "Remember to pick some long ones and plenty of berries," she instructs us.

We are filled with memories of picking the greens and making the wreaths for Christmas. Holidays and traditions make memories that last, even with Alzheimer's disease.

"Donald called to say he's coming home for a visit," I report. "He read our manuscript and decided to come now, rather than wait until July."

My parents are thrilled. I was surprised myself when my brother Donald called late one night from the West. We talked for an hour, the longest call ever. Donald wanted to know all about my "Fridays with Susie." He wanted to understand the changes in our mother's life. Most of all, he wanted to be here, with her, now.

After our walk we settle in on the couch with a cup of tea and begin taping. The sun peeks through the clouds, dancing on the yellow poplar leaves amidst the gray bark of the bare maple trees. The view of the mountains is muted now. Autumn is winding down. Our story is nearing the end.

I start by asking my mother how she is feeling this week.

I forgot four things this morning on our way out to your house. But it doesn't matter. I'll bring them another time.

I made fourteen gallons of applesauce to freeze for the winter. We can bring it to Jackson for the kids' breakfast!

Once again, I am surprised by Susie's world. She can organize herself to make fourteen gallons of applesauce, yet she forgot four things in one morning on her way out the door.

Susie is pleased to report on her speech last night as a former president of the World Affairs Council at the director's retirement dinner. She started right out with her disarming candor:

I have Alzheimer's. Otherwise, I would go on for half an hour about how wonderful Dave Larsen has been for thirty-five years!

Everyone laughed right along with her, through their tears, relieved to share her joy and her sorrow.

I ask my mother how she first became involved with the World Affairs Council, back in the early 1960s.

I was interested in world affairs way back then. We invited foreign students to stay at our house when you kids were young. I enjoyed having foreign guests, so the World Affairs Council would call whenever someone interesting came to New Hampshire. I had the most beautiful house and a nice guest room, so they came to stay with us. Then when I was in the legislature, I would bring the foreign visitors to see the State House.

The World Affairs Council brought in famous speakers and held conferences. Secretary of State Dean Rusk came to our house for cocktails before his speech. New Hampshire had the first presidential primary, so everyone came to visit here first! Later, I organized a big conference on China before President Nixon went there.

Now I am flooded with memories. I remember at age five showing students from Martinique and Guadeloupe how to use a dishwasher. Who could forget the night Dean Rusk came to visit, when Daddy confronted the Secret Service men on our front lawn as he ran to a neighbor's house to get the right whiskey for our distinguished guest. I vividly recall a huge red dragon in the middle of our dining room table with all the materials for the conference on "Red China." Foreign policy was a constant theme in our family.

Malcolm digresses for a moment to tell the story of his parents' trip to San Francisco to attend the international conference that led to the creation of the United Nations in April 1945. My father was a nineteen-year-old fighter pilot in World War II. After flying seventy-two missions, he was shot down during the Battle of the Bulge, two days before Christmas 1944.

As Malcolm is telling the story, Susie breaks out in song, to the tune of "Why Do I Love You?":

> *December twenty-third,*
> *That was all we heard.*
> *Was it your parachute?*
> *Info was mute.*
> *April's news that the Krauts held you*
> *Made our gray skies turn a bright blue.*

I am intrigued once again by my mother's memory. How can she remember the words to a family song written sixty years ago, but not what she ate for breakfast this morning?

Susie was just fifteen when Malcolm was shot down, but she clearly remembers her sister Mary coming home from skiing with the McLanes at Cannon Mountain. Mary burst into tears as she told her family about the terrible news that Malcolm had been shot down and was missing in action in Germany. Apparently, Judge and Elisabeth felt that going skiing was the best way to cope with their shock and sorrow.

For many months, my grandparents thought that their youngest son had died in battle. In fact, he had been captured and held as a prisoner of war in Germany.

Judge and Elisabeth learned of Malcolm's survival in April, just as they boarded the train in Montreal bound for the West to attend the historic conference. In San Francisco my grandfather was the first Dartmouth trustee to interview Assistant Secretary of State John Dickey, who became the next president of the college. With hope in their hearts after months of grieving, my grandparents sought peace in the world through the creation of the United Nations at the end of World War II.

As the news this week focuses on the war on terrorism at home and abroad, I am curious about my parents' travels and their commitment to understanding world affairs. My mother and father take turns talking as they slowly piece together their lifelong itinerary. Susie begins.

Our first travel across the country was to visit Sally in Squaw Valley each winter for three years leading up to the 1960 Olympics. We took Robin and Donald with us in 1959. They loved to ski! Malcolm was chairman of the Olympic Ski Committee, so we went to all the Olympics and FIS World Championships back then. We went to Squaw Valley in 1960, Chamonix in 1962, and Innsbruck in 1964.

Then when you kids were young, we drove out West one summer to visit Sally's family and our ski friends in Helena, Montana. A few years later, we took you kids to Europe. We drove around for six weeks in a VW bus for the Grand Tour! For several years after that we were paying college tuitions, so we didn't travel as much.

Then Malcolm picks up the travelogue:

Susie's first big foreign trip was in 1972 to Japan as a guest of the Japanese government. The group was selected as "up-and-coming" political leaders, including Dick Thornburgh, who became governor of Pennsylvania and U.S. attorney general, and others who served in state legislatures, in the Carter administration and as vice president of Harvard.

Susie adds her own memories:

I can remember that Japan was just so unusual, day after day. The first night we were in the hotel bar during an earthquake. We went to Hiroshima, too. I invited them all to Newfound Lake for a reunion that summer. I called them my Japanese friends. We stayed in touch for a long time. Dick and

Ginny Thornburgh came to visit every summer for years as their kids were growing up.

During the 1980s we skied in Europe every winter with Penny Pitou, who we knew from the Squaw Valley Olympics. Then we went to Europe for three months when Malcolm had a sabbatical from his law firm, sailing in Scotland and traveling through England, France, Hungary, and Greece.

Then Malcolm picks up the litany of travels:

In 1989, Susie went with a legislative delegation to Korea. Then in 1991, she went to South Africa on a political trip to meet with the leaders of all the various racial factions.

Susie adds:

It was fascinating!

Malcolm continues:

In 1994, we went around the world when Susie retired from the Legislature. You and Zachary joined us in Scotland at the beginning of the trip.

Susie chimes in:

I read the journal the other day with the pictures of Zach in Scotland. We went to France, Spain, Greece, Israel, Kenya, India, Nepal, Thailand, Australia, New Zealand, and then home via Hawaii to see Sally in California.

I am intrigued by my parents' lifelong ambition to see the world and understand foreign cultures. Their worldview led our entire family to travel and explore foreign lands and cultures.

Robin and Marion visited cousins in India and Thailand, then later traveled to Kenya to work in a rural health clinic. Donald and his family spent several winters living on the beach in Mexico, soaking in the sun and local culture. Debbie and Peter lived in Spain for a year when their girls were young, then skied in South America several summers.

Alan's daughter Laura is learning Japanese and will study in Japan soon. His daughter Carrie took a school trip to Paris and plans to return to travel in Europe during college.

When I worked for Congressman Pete McCloskey, we toured Lebanon, Syria, and Israel with a congressional delegation in 1979. Then I spent six weeks in Zimbabwe, Mozambique, and South Africa in 1980, studying race relations, emerging independence, and the devastating impact of apartheid, just as my mother did ten years later.

Susie loves revisiting her journals and talking about all our foreign trips. Today our conversation turns to the news this week that Pakistani scientists may have passed secrets about nuclear weapons to Osama bin Laden. My father tells the story of my uncle Dave Bradley, who wrote a book about the atomic bomb called *No Place to Hide*:

> *Dave Bradley was in medical school in the Army during World War II. In 1946, he was sent to the Bikini Atoll in the Pacific, where the first postwar atom bomb tests were taking place. Americans were so naïve about atomic energy and nuclear power. We just didn't understand yet how dangerous it was. Later they stopped testing bombs above ground because of what they learned from these tests.*
>
> *Dave was a radiation officer out there. He was supposed to go aboard the ships after the tests to see if they were safe. I don't think he ever thought they were safe, but they passed whatever exposure was allowed. A lot of troops probably were exposed to radiation.*
>
> *Dave kept a journal of his experience. When he came back to the medical internship world, he was so horrified that nobody gave a damn about the bomb tests. He published his journal in a magazine, and later as a book called* No Place to Hide.

The book was a very straightforward account of the Bikini atom bomb tests which appalled people who were worried about the destruction of atomic weapons. As a medical doctor, Dave made some honest comments about the impact of radiation. He became involved with the World Federalist Organization promoting world peace. Dave spoke all over the country about what happened on the Bikini Islands and how inappropriate it was to be developing nuclear bombs.

My mother and I listen intently to my father's story. Then I ask, "How about you, Momma, what do you think about the current threat to world peace?"

I don't think about it at all. . . . I read the front page of the paper and then, that's it. [She smiles.]

As the world comes to terms with the threat of war and the ultimate fear of terrorists with access to nuclear bombs, I realize that my mother can simply tune out terror. Is this the silver lining of Alzheimer's disease? In Susie's world, there is no place to hide from the destruction within her brain. Bioterrorism at home or war halfway around the world is just front-page news. Nothing more, nothing less.

Slowly I realize that I have the same choice. Live in fear or simply come to terms with our changing world. President George W. Bush said this week, "we have refused to live in a state of panic, or a state of denial." His words ring true.

Anthrax, Afghanistan, Alzheimer's. I realize that in my life, it's all the same state of mind.

CHAPTER TWENTY-ONE

MIND, MEMORY, AND AGING

NOVEMBER SINKS INTO our psyche slowly, as the leaves gather on the ground and the wind whistles through the bare trees. The chill settles into our bones. The clear, cold nights seep into our hearts and minds. Winter is coming. We rake leaves and stack wood for the fire. Wool is our protection now, soft and warm against our skin.

Planting bulbs is my harbinger of hope. Daffodils and tulips buried in the ground hold secrets of spring. Even on days when the wind blows and the temperature drops, the setting sun lights up the western sky with a kaleidoscope of colors, brilliant yellow, peach, and pink around a blazing red ball of fire.

My mother's life settles into the season, softly slipping away into gray, with sudden bursts of brightness. Somehow the very process of recording her life story and reading it, chapter by chapter, refreshes her memory.

Now Susie holds forth over dinner with old friends, telling her story, line by line, verse by verse, as though she is reading from a book. Then she pauses, searching for the right words, and says with a smile, "I have Alzheimer's, so I don't remember the rest."

My parents call to report in on another adventure. They visited The Birches, the new assisted living community in Concord that specializes in memory loss, just across the road from St. Paul's School.

"I love it," Susie says, sounding like a teenager visiting boarding school, about to begin the next chapter in her life.

"It's perfect! Malcolm can come visit anytime. We can even go out for a drive or to dinner in town whenever we want," she reports.

My mother sounds excited, as if she is surprised by the relative freedom. My father is pleased, too, as though he is relieved to have a plan for their future.

"We'll ask if Susie can have a bird feeder in the yard," Malcolm says with a laugh. "That will make her happy."

⨎

On Thursday, I drive to Hanover for dinner with my aunt Lilla at Kendal. Then we attend a forum at Dartmouth by three leading medical scholars on "Mind, Memory, and Aging: Perspectives on Preventing Memory Loss and Alzheimer's Disease."

Dr. Robert Santulli, assistant professor of psychiatry at Dartmouth Medical School and president of the Alzheimer's Association of Vermont and New Hampshire, cuts right to the chase in his opening remarks: noting "We simply do not have the medical knowledge or technology to prevent Alzheimer's disease."

Twenty thousand people in New Hampshire have Alzheimer's now. Age is the number one risk factor. The risk of

Alzheimer's is 10 percent over age sixty-five, rising to 50 percent by age eighty-five. With the aging population, the risk of Alzheimer's is increasing exponentially.

As Dr. Santulli reviews the other risk factors, my focus shifts from my mother to my own life for the very first time. Beyond age, gender is a factor. Women are more likely than men to have Alzheimer's, largely because there are more older women than men in the population. Genetics plays an important role, too. The risk increases two to four times if a close blood relative has the disease.

The one "glimmer of hope" is that behavior modification might delay the onset of memory loss and Alzheimer's disease. As Dr. Santulli speaks, I think about my mother, checking off the factors on his list that may have contributed to her decline. Then I think about my own health and lifestyle choices. Looking up and down the rows of white hair and wrinkled faces, I realize that everyone in the auditorium shares just one thought this evening: "Am I too late to change?"

While describing the list of "behaviors that have been associated with Alzheimer's through scientific research," Dr. Santulli emphasizes that "no conclusion can be reached to prove the cause of memory loss or Alzheimer's disease at this stage of medical knowledge."

Although there are many potential risk factors for Alzheimer's disease or other dementias, the results of scientific research thus far point to alcohol use, brain injury, education, level of social engagement, marital status, level of activity, and exercise as potential indicators of the risk of memory loss and Alzheimer's disease.

The medical research from around the world is fascinating. Studies from France suggest that moderate use of red wine may decrease the risk, presumably due to the effect of antioxidants. But everyone seems to agree that long-term alcohol abuse significantly increases the risk. On the other hand, smoking may actually decrease the risk because, as Dr. Santulli notes with a smile, early death leaves less chance of Alzheimer's.

Education may lower the risk, either by creating a "cognitive reserve" of brain cells or by stimulating the synapses, which are the connectors that form the neural pathways in the brain. One study shows that each year of higher education results in a 17 percent lower chance of Alzheimer's. But, Dr. Santulli points out, the research may be flawed because people with more education and higher social and economic status often do well on cognitive tests, thereby masking the effects of the disease.

Numerous studies from New Haven to Stockholm conclude that social isolation significantly increases the risk of cognitive decline. Similarly, research in Greece and France demonstrates that marriage reduces the risk. More studies conclude that increasing the time devoted to intellectual activities or exercise decreases the risk of Alzheimer's disease.

Following his review of the behavioral risk factors, Dr. Santulli introduces a list of possible medical interventions. The news of the week is a breakthrough study of ibuprofen in mice, resulting in an 80 percent reduction in plaque formation in the brains of mice. Although the results are stunning, Dr. Santulli is cautious, noting the high dosage of ibuprofen in the study. Scientists must continue to probe the impact of anti-inflammatory drugs to fully understand whether Motrin, Advil, or ibuprofen may delay the onset of memory loss and Alzheimer's disease.

Antioxidants, such as vitamin E, may also slow the progression of Alzheimer's disease. Dr. Santulli lists foods high in antioxidants, including blueberries, strawberrries, raisins, carrots, tomatoes, and spinach.

An alternative remedy sold in health food stores known as *Ginkgo biloba* have been shown to have a small effect on retaining cognitive function. While acknowledging that medical science has yet to discover the definitive prevention, cure, or treatment of Alzheimer's disease, Dr. Santulli holds out hope with his faith in scientific research.

Dr. Julie Fago, associate professor of community and family medicine at Dartmouth, focuses her remarks on women with Alzheimer's, beginning with the very first patient ever diagnosed with the disease in 1901. Dr. Fago describes research on why women are three times more likely than men to develop Alzheimer's.

Studies have shown that women treated with hormone replacement therapy, namely estrogen, demonstrate higher cognitive testing. Mice treated with estrogen perform better in mazes. Future scientific discovery may confirm a role for estrogen to delay the onset of Alzheimer's.

Closing her remarks with a quote from George Eliot, "It's never too late to be who you might have been," Dr. Fago concurs with Dr. Santulli's advice to "use it or lose it." Physical and mental exercise, as well as a satisfying social life, still offers the best prevention for memory loss and Alzheimer's disease. Besides, she adds brightly, "it's a better way to live!"

Dr. David Knopman, a neurologist at the Mayo Clinic and a professor of neurology, outlines the recent dramatic advances in the scientific understanding of Alzheimer's. In his closing remarks, Dr. Knopman describes the cholinesterase inhibitors, Aricept and Exelon, which have proved to delay the onset of memory loss and Alzheimer's disease.

Lilla and I are intrigued by his description of the criteria used to diagnose Alzheimer's disease—namely, "memory loss and impaired daily functioning resulting in dependence on others for assistance."

Many believe that a definitive diagnosis of Alzheimer's cannot be confirmed until the autopsy, a grim Catch-22 for patients and their families. Research reveals, however, that experienced physicians are accurate 90 percent of the time with a diagnosis based on the patient's personal history, a medical exam, and a process of ruling out other known causes of memory loss and declining cognitive function.

Lilla and I are fascinated by the presentation. As I leave, my aunt gives me a large envelope filled with articles about Alzheimer's. On the back she has written a note: "I want copies of anything you find helpful for my family in the future."

Even as we dedicate our lives to "mental and physical exercise and a satisfying social network," Lilla and I realize that there is no place to hide from memory loss and Alzheimer's. Medical science knows no prevention, no cure, and no treatment.

We refuse to live in a state of panic, or in a state of denial. We will live in Susie's world, appreciating our lives in the moment, with faith in the future of scientific research. Patience is a virtue. Peace of mind is our reward.

༃

Driving home on the dark, lonely highway, thinking about the road ahead, the future sinks into my heart, through the blues rhythms of Eva Cassidy, singing from her soul:

> *Heaven,*
> *I'm in Heaven,*
> *and my heart beats so*
> *that I can hardly speak,*
> *and I seem to find*
> *the happiness I seek,*
> *when we're out together*
> *dancing cheek to cheek.*

I stare out into the cold, clear night, watching the stars sparkling in the heavens above. I smile as I think about my time this fall with my mother, our last dance together, as I sing along.

CHAPTER TWENTY-TWO

THE NINTH AND TENTH FRIDAYS: 'TIS A GIFT TO BE SIMPLE'

THE LEAVES HAVE fallen from the trees. The first snowflakes flutter in the air. Susie makes her partridge berry wreaths and plans our Thanksgiving dinner. The holidays will soon be upon us once again.

On Friday morning, I take my mother shopping at JC Penney's for new clothes. Lately she seems to wear the same outfits over and over. I finally realize that she has not been shopping for herself since she left the legislature. In the beginning, she was being frugal, but now I know that my mother can't manage clothes shopping on her own.

As we drive to the mall, she says to me, "I can't even imagine living another ten years."

I've become used to my mother's openness, but now I am the one who is at a loss for words. I sit silently, searching for the right words to respond to her.

"I understand how you feel, Momma, but you do have a good life right now, don't you think?" I ask cautiously.

"Yes, I do now," she says, then pauses. "But I don't want to live for another ten years." She smiles at me. "I'm tired of reading the paper every morning and such."

My mother enjoys our shopping spree, as long as we keep it simple. She is easy to please, if you find what she likes to wear. While we carefully peruse the racks of clothes, my mother announces that she doesn't wear black. We find several bright red tops to wear over gray and blue slacks and a pair of comfortable blue shoes. She is happy with her purchases, like a child opening birthday presents.

Susie slowly signs her name on the credit card slip. Then she thanks me for coming shopping with her. We both know that shopping for new clothes is one more thing that she can no longer manage alone.

Then we stop by Home Depot for the narcissus bulbs to plant for an annual tradition of Christmas cheer in Susie's world. My mother has never been to Home Depot. She is overcome by the warehouse filled with all the stuff of modern living. Susie wanders up and down the aisles like a child, gazing at the shelves overflowing with modern conveniences of every shape and kind. I realize that my mother is past needing the endless variety of material possessions, but she is delighted with the narcissus bulbs. Susie recognizes hope and inspiration in her world.

Monday night, Debbie calls to report on her visit over the weekend with Susie. My sister is learning to give her time to respond in a conversation. "I bit my tongue to let her talk," Debbie says with a laugh. We both realize that Susie knows what she wants to say most of the time, but we only have a fifty-fifty chance of being right if we fill in the words for her. If we're wrong, then she gets even more confused.

Later in the week, I accompany my mother to her doctor's appointment. The nurse confirms that her pulse and blood pressure are excellent. Her physical health is remarkably good, despite her weight and lack of exercise.

Then the nurse reviews Susie's bag of medications, checking the dosage against the list in her medical record on the computer. As I watch, the nurse asks my mother over and over again, "How often do you take this? What's the dosage? How many milligrams?" Susie is patient, but somewhat baffled by the questions.

When the nurse gets to the vitamins and supplements, she begins asking over and over, "Why are you taking this one?"

Susie answers, patiently and politely, "I have no idea why, but the man in the pharmacy told me to take it. . . . So I do."

The final list is impressive, a complete account of all the various preventions and treatments currently under study by medical researchers around the world. Three times a day, every day, my mother takes a handful of pills for memory loss, including Advil, Exelon, *Ginkgo biloba*, melatonin, and vitamin E.

She also takes aspirin to avoid another stroke, as well as several medications for various maladies and to help her sleep at night. Susie is a walking, talking medical experiment, taking her pills without question, with complete faith in her health care providers.

When Dr. Vanderlinde walks into the room, my mother lights up. Susie is wearing her new bright red top, with plenty of red lipstick. She announces to her doctor, "We went shopping at J.C. Penney's. I wore this for you!"

Tanya is warm and kind to my mother, asking her how she is feeling.

*I'm just fine. . . . But I can't remember anything anymore.
. . . And I can't taste anything either* [Susie says with a smile].

*I went to the bank this morning to get money from the
machine. But I couldn't remember the number, so I couldn't get
the money. I tried every number I knew, but none of them
worked.*

*Then I went into the bank to ask the man, but he said that
they didn't know my number either. When I told Malcolm, he
said that he would give me the money.*

*This is my daughter, Annie. She is my replacement. . . . I
can't remember anything and Malcolm is being so nice about
it. . . . But I can still cook, and do the laundry and all the
driving, as long as Malcolm is the navigator.*

When my mother mentions that she can't sleep at night,
Tanya asks about whether she naps in the afternoon. Their discussion about balancing daytime napping with nighttime
sleeping reminds me of the same dilemma with a four year old
child. I realize that the analogy between Alzheimer's disease and
raising a child in reverse is coming true in Susie's world.

Tanya reviews my mother's medical record, describing to us
the neuro-psych testing by the Department of Psychiatry at
Dartmouth in May 2001. The doctor describes my mother's most
recent MRI findings, noting "global atrophy in the frontal lobe"
of her brain. Tanya confirms to us that her "memory difficulties
and functional loss meet the criteria for a diagnosis of
Alzheimer's disease."

My mother's acceptance of her doctor's confirmation of the
Alzheimer's diagnosis reminds me of her approach all her life to
the news of another pregnancy. *"And so, there it was."*

Susie responds to her doctor, "I made a speech to the World
Affairs Council. I told them all that I have Alzheimer's, otherwise
I would talk for half an hour!"

On her way out the door, Tanya reminds my mother to cut back on alcohol and to switch the melatonin to the evening, or even take a Sominex, to help her sleep. Then the doctor asks my mother to make an appointment to see her in six months. When she says good-bye, my mother adds cheerily, "We're going to Egypt in January. I don't care if it is dangerous. Everyone has to die sometime!"

৵

Thursday night my parents come over for dinner with my nephew Erik, who is visiting from the West. Susie cooks a delicious dinner, lemon chicken with rice, then serves Starbucks mocha chip ice cream for dessert. She is still a tough act to follow in the kitchen.

When I offer to divulge to Erik the secret to finding and keeping a girlfriend, Zach grabs pen and paper to write down the magic. Everyone listens attentively, as I explain that what a woman wants in life is a man who will talk with her and listen to her. Pandemonium breaks loose!

"Oh, Annie, give him something feasible at least," Brad says, as everyone laughs.

Later, as Susie and Brad finish the dishes, Malcolm talks to Erik and me about how she is doing this week.

"Susie hardly reads at all anymore, but yesterday she was reading ahead in one of the Alzheimer's books. She came to a section about the final stage, when total memory loss and confusion sets in. Susie brought it to me and pointed out the paragraph about the final stage. She wanted me to read it, but she was still smiling, almost as though she didn't really comprehend how bad it could be at the end."

My father's eyes fill with tears. "I told her, 'We'll get through it together, Susie, you and me.' "

I am utterly amazed at how far my father has come this fall. He is a new man, totally open and honest with his feelings and able to communicate with our family in a whole new way. We are all blessed to be together, to have each other, and most of all, to find one another this way.

ॐ

On Friday morning, Susie arrives at my house with Erik, who is planning to videotape our final interview. The sun streams in through the windows, as we settle in on the couch with our coffee and begin taping.

My mother is having a good day. Her thoughts are coherent, even though the words are often hard to come by. As we talk about her defection from Republican to Democrat over the original gender gap in American politics, she says,

> I can't get over what's happening in Afghanistan, how the people are coming back out in the streets. The women have gone back to work and to their lives.
>
> I think that that is the essence of my life. I went to the legislature at age forty and I sat down next to Betty Green. I didn't realize until that point, having grown up at Dartmouth and married Malcolm, who was a Rhodes scholar, that women were as bright as men. That was the most incredible experience of my life.

We talk about New Hampshire politics heating up for the 2002 election, with major races among Republicans and Democrats for the U.S. Senate, Congress, and governor. My mother is pleased to be supporting another woman for governor, her friend and former Senate colleague Bev Hollingworth.

Then she holds forth once again on the tax structure of the State of New Hampshire. My mother's only regret in her political career was never passing an income tax to support public education. Now she wants to write an editorial for the newspaper about why New Hampshire needs an income tax, but she is having trouble grasping the details for her argument. I offer to help, knowing that she still cares deeply about the future of our state.

Our final taping session winds down with Erik filming the two of us, mother and daughter, talking on the couch about our lives. We both want to make the world a better place. We both care about our families and our communities, from the children of New Hampshire to the women of Afghanistan.

"How have you felt about our time talking together this fall?" I ask.

I have enjoyed it completely! Looking at that picture of you and Jeanne Shaheen, our first woman Governor, I feel very strongly that women have come far in seventy-two years. When I was young, growing up at Dartmouth, there were no women. Then you went to Dartmouth, in the third class of women. I cannot get over the fact that you are a lawyer.

"What do you think about our time together this fall taping the story of your life?" I ask.

I think that doing this with you is the cause of me being positive, instead of negative, about Alzheimer's. I look back on my life and I just feel wonderful.

"Do you think that the process of talking about your feelings has helped you cope with Alzheimer's?" I wonder.

Yes, I do. I can't talk any more about the present. . . . [pause] Malcolm and I are going to go to Egypt, but I can't remember where we're going. I know I will enjoy it, wherever it is! . . . So that's it.

"Are you worried about whether it's safe with what's going on in the world?" I ask.

No, because if it's not safe, I'll die early. . . . I am into reading about Alzheimer's. It discourages me so about the later stages, incontinence and that sort of thing . . . not tasting, not remembering. You are in bed the last year or so. I get depressed by that.

"The only saving grace to this disease is that when you get to that stage, you won't realize it," I say softly. "We will be there to make you comfortable, to keep you happy living in the moment." I smile, trying to reassure my mother and myself about what the future holds for us.

My mother is smiling now, too. Once again I am trying to balance reality with hope and compassion. I want to share my mother's candor without breaking her heart, or mine.

"But if you go out in a hijacking in Egypt, we'll wish you well," I say. "At least you and Daddy will be together!"

My mother laughs, then continues sharing her thoughts about life now.

Malcolm is so unusual about the illness. He is really wonderful. He is getting older, too . . . five years older than I am. He doesn't ski anymore since he had his knees done. . . . He is very kind now. He's gone back to where he was when he married me because I was a young girl.

"He has read the Alzheimer's books, too." I say. "Now he is much more open talking about his feelings. Daddy is so loyal to you and fond of you. He loves you very much, don't you think?" I ask expectantly.

Susie is smiling now and her eyes are twinkling as she responds.

He really does love me . . . [She pauses, smiling as she searches for the words.] I love him very much, too. I feel that he is kinder now . . . It's nice . . . it's very nice. . . . In fact, it's excellent!

I give my mother a hug and lay my head on her shoulder. "I love you, Momma," I say softly.

I love you, too. Your sisters are into their own life . . . and you are into mine!

"That's what I keep saying about why you love the book. It's about you!" We laugh as our time together today comes to an end.

ॐ

Looking back on my "Fridays with Susie" this fall, I am reminded of the Shaker song that we sang at our wedding, "Simple Gifts,"

> *'Tis a gift to be simple*
> *'Tis a gift to be free,*
> *'Tis a gift*
> *to come down where we ought to be,*
> *And when we find ourselves*
> *In the place just right,*
> *'Twill be in the valley*
> *of love and delight.*

One by one, week by week, I have felt my mother's life lessons sink into my life. There are no strangers in my world now, just folks I haven't met yet. I am living in the moment and finding joy in simple pleasures. I am learning to let the memory of misery fade first. I am appreciating the natural beauty of the land—lakes, mountains, and sky. I am reaching out to family and friends, opening my heart and soul, laughing together over joy and crying together over sorrow. I am learning to live by not being afraid to die.

I realize now that my life is my own life to live. Everyone has different memories of our family. Our perception becomes our own reality. No matter what I accomplish, I will always be the youngest child in our family; yet I have no regrets about the choices I made or the decisions that framed my life.

I know now that others in my family have made different choices. In the end, that's what life is all about. My mother has no regrets about the choices she made over the course of her long and meaningful life. Now all we have to do is listen carefully to hear her wisdom, to find peace in our world and faith in our hearts.

ॐ

On Sunday, I walk and talk again with Lucia, who recently visited her parents in Maine. The visit went well. Lucia is pleased that our conversations have helped her accept her mother's Alzheimer's and appreciate each glimmer of recognition and hope. Whenever Lucia left the room, her mother's face would light up when she returned. She would say, "Lucia, so wonderful to see you!" Her soul may be lost, but her heart is found.

As we say good-bye, Lucia says to me, "One of the hardest parts of coping with Alzheimer's is that you never know when to grieve." Her words comfort me later in the evening. Soaking in the hot tub with the moonlight drifting through the trees, the tears begin to flow, hot on my cheeks.

Half of the grief about Alzheimer's is letting go. Learning to let go may be the last lesson I learn from my mother.

Patience is a virtue. Peace in my heart is the reward.

PART TWO

SPRING 2004

CHAPTER TWENTY-THREE

HEAVEN'S GATE

CHANGE IS THE ONLY constant in our lives. Slowly, day by day, week by week, my mother is slipping away from us all. Grief comes in waves, at the sight of a flock of geese flying south or a child skating on the ice. Memories fill my mind. Loss fills my heart.

The snow is soft and deep. The world is white all around as I drive into town, past The Birches, past the hospital, past the hospice house. The tall pines are drooping from the weight of the storm. Snow clings to the branches. The sky is filled with white as the snow drifts down in fluffy flakes. The world is all white, a cocoon of soft, downy flakes. I am in Heaven. The tears flow freely down my cheeks. Susie will be safe here, far from the cares of the world.

Heaven,
I'm in Heaven,
And my heart beats so
That I can hardly speak,
And I seem to find
The happiness I seek,
When we're out together
Dancing cheek to cheek.

First, there is the beginning. Then, there is the end. Everything else is in the middle. Facing Alzheimer's disease is about coming to terms with living in the middle, in limbo, in a constant state of change. We are living the last dance, feeling the anticipation that the party will end, yet hoping that the feeling of love in our hearts will last forever.

Three winters have come and gone in our lives since my "Fridays with Susie." Life goes on, adjusting day by day to the changes all around us, but the music never stops. Children grow up, parents age. The leaves fall off the trees, the snow and ice come again. The cycle of life goes on, one season at a time.

The Last Dance has become a metaphor for a life worth living. My mother reads her book cover to cover every day. Then she begins at the beginning again. She loves sharing her story. For many months now, reading the story of her life over and over again, Susie has held on to her identity, even as the person within her slips away.

We have all savored our last dance together, each of us coming to terms with Alzheimer's disease in our own way. We live in the present with Susie, entering her time zone whenever we visit. We leave our cares at the door, focusing instead on the moment when her face lights up and she smiles, waiting for a kiss on both cheeks. Every glimmer of recognition is a gift from the past. Every moment together is a memory for the future. We stand at Heaven's Gate, waiting, hoping, praying for peace in our hearts and in her soul.

CHAPTER TWENTY-FOUR

'LIVE FREE OR DIE'

*M*Y PARENTS CONTINUED on with their
busy life for as long as possible, despite Alzheimer's disease and
the challenges facing my mother. In 2002, they traveled to Egypt
in January and to France in the fall, enjoying the culture and the
company of their group. I remember worrying about Susie as I
dropped them off at the airport, watching her trail behind
Malcolm, wandering through the busy crowd. But my father was
patient and they persevered.

In June 2002, my mother's older sister, Mary Kilmarx, died
very suddenly of a stroke. In their retirement, Bob and Mary
were living a full and active life, skiing in the winter out West
and planning a hiking trip to Norway in the summer. Then one
Saturday evening, Mary went to the hospital after a minor stroke
left her speech impaired but her mind alert. She worked on the
Sunday *New York Times* crossword puzzle in the morning. She

even remembered my parents' phone number when Bob called them with the news.

By Sunday evening, when Bob and their daughter Elizabeth left to go home, Mary wondered aloud, "Who's going to give me a ride home?"

"We'll come back in the morning to pick you up," they said reassuringly.

But Mary died the next day from a massive stroke. Everyone was stunned. Instead of leaving to go hiking in Norway, Bob began organizing a memorial celebration to honor Mary's life.

We grieved together over the loss of Mary's incredible energy and enthusiasm for life. Family and friends gathered to honor her indelible spirit and her many accomplishments. Mary lived a long and meaningful life, but her sudden loss left everyone feeling more vulnerable.

My mother graciously accepted her older sister's peaceful death. When Susie spoke with her cousin, Alan Hall, after Mary's death, she said simply, "I just feel that she is in Heaven now."

As our family slowly comes to terms with losing our mother one day at a time, we are constantly reminded that life and death come and go on their own terms. No one decides how or when our loved ones will die. Whenever I look into my mother's sparkling Neidlinger eyes, I think of her sisters and of my cousins coming to terms with losing their mothers to cancer or a sudden stroke. We did not choose our mother's slow demise, but we know we have time to say good-bye, over and over again.

༄

In the summer of 2002, Brad and I took our boys, Zach and Travis, on a camping trip out West. We stayed a week with our Hudson cousins on Lake Tahoe, mountain biking and swimming during the day and reminiscing late into the night about our mothers, the Neidlinger twins.

When they were young, Susan and Sally were called "Sue-Sal" by their father because he could not tell them apart. Now our stories about growing up in New Hampshire and California are entwined like strands of DNA, with a genetic link that spans three thousand miles for a lifetime of interwoven memories.

Our mothers were so similar that once when Susie called from New Hampshire, my cousin Bill said to her over the telephone, "Mom, I thought you were in the kitchen!" We often joke that we are closer to siblings than cousins because we share half our genes. Everyone laughs about the time my cousin Jake appeared in our Christmas card as a stand-in for my brother Donald.

Laughing together helps us cope with the loss in our hearts. Slowly, day by day, we are learning to let go of the past and to prepare for the future. We are learning to live our own lives by not being afraid to die.

જ

Our camping trip continued on to British Columbia and the spectacular scenery of the Canadian Rockies in Lake Louise and Banff. Brad and I tackled the challenging mountain biking terrain with Zach and Travis leading the way. At the end of our trip, we stayed with Donald and his family in the North Cascades of central Washington. My brother is an avid mountain biker, too. Our boys loved exploring the wooded trails and mountain peaks with their uncle.

Everyone enjoyed catching up with the cousins. Erik has moved back to Lake Tahoe. Karissa is in college in Bellingham. Abi holds down the fort at home, playing volleyball and living the teenage life. They marvel at Zach, who grew a foot in a year and a half, while Travis is not far behind. Change is the only constant in our lives. Life goes on, sharing stories, making memories, living in the moment, one day at a time.

In July, my parents landed in Seattle the day we flew back East. I taught my father to drive our new van in the airport parking lot. Then off they went for one last big adventure on their own. Looking back, we are amazed at their fortitude and good fortune that summer.

My parents drove four thousand miles together, from Seattle to New Hampshire, visiting family and friends along the way. They even went to the Ski Hall of Fame in Ishpeming, Michigan, where my aunt Sally and my father are honored.

They eventually arrived home in August, pulling into our driveway in Hopkinton, enthused and exhausted.

"I drove most of the way," Susie announced with a big smile.

Malcolm explained how well she drove for long stretches of highway, so he could rest. They enjoyed the trip and their time together on the road.

"We only had one problem," he said.

"What was that?" I asked anxiously.

"Well, at the Canadian border, when the guard asked if we had any contraband, Susie said, Yes, and I said, No," he explained.

"What happened?" I asked, vividly imagining the scene. The uncertainty of our two worlds was colliding, with the heightened tension of terrorism at the border and the shifting reality of Alzheimer's in my mother's mind.

"Oh, he realized that she was confused and he let us go," Malcolm said with a laugh. "But it was a close call."

Life is full of confusion and close calls these days. We all feel more vulnerable, but my parents refuse to live in a state of panic, or in a state of denial. They live free in Susie's world, appreciating life in the moment, aware of the threat but focused on the opportunity. Safety and security are on our minds. Peace is in our hearts.

֍

Passion, patience and perseverance best describe my parents' life together since Alzheimer's disease entered their world. I am reminded of my mother's philosophy facing the early death of her twin sister, Sally.

One of the best things that ever happened to me was to be with Sally before she died. I couldn't do anything about her dying, except to be there with her. I have discovered that half of the grief about death is guilt. I didn't have any guilt when Sally died. I stayed with her for two and a half months. When she died I wasn't sad.

For two and a half years since our "Fridays with Susie," my father has devoted his life to caring for my mother, twenty-four hours a day, seven days a week, day in and day out. Over time, their life slowly settled into a comfortable routine. Every morning, they watched *The Today Show* while Malcolm served Susie breakfast in bed — a banana and muffin with a cup of coffee.

After breakfast, a home health aide from the Visiting Nurse Association came to bathe Susie and help with the laundry and cleaning, while Malcolm went to the office. A distinguished trusts and estates lawyer for over fifty years at Orr and Reno, my father appreciates the company of his colleagues and the routine of his clients and accounts now more than ever before.

At noon, my father came home every day to serve lunch, a bowl of soup with yogurt for dessert. After lunch, my parents took a nap and then went for a drive, enjoying the sights of scenic New Hampshire. Occasionally, they went out to dinner at their favorite restaurant, but most nights Malcolm served dinner at home. As time went by, he became a fan of Boston Market for healthy takeout dinners.

Every evening at six o'clock, they watched the news on *McNeil-Lehrer*. Then they watched a movie before settling in for the night. As time passed, my father would get up in the night several times to help my mother to the bathroom. Everyone, especially my mother, marveled at his patience and kindness.

"Malcolm is so kind to me now," she would say with a smile.

"I love you, Susie," he would say, tears in his eyes, "and I will be here for you."

Friends and family came to visit, staying for lunch or tea by the fire. As the months passed, Susie spoke fewer and fewer words, but she always managed to say her favorite line:

"I have Alzheimer's. I can't speak, but I listen to your every word."

The loss of speech is called aphasia, meaning "partial or total loss of the ability to speak or comprehend speech, resulting from brain damage." Day by day, week by week, we learned to accept the changes in our mother's life. One by one, we learned from Susie that we cannot do anything about aging and Alzheimer's disease, except to be there for her and for each other. The New Hampshire state motto emblazoned on every license plate is *Live Free or Die*. My parents are learning to live free in the moment, to find joy in the simple pleasures of life, to be there for one another.

In the end, we all will die one day. Until then, we are learning to appreciate what is left of my mother's life, not to dwell on what is lost. Overcoming the grief of Alzheimer's disease is about learning to be there, to savor our time together. That's why we call it the present. It's a gift that keeps on giving, one day at a time.

CHAPTER TWENTY-FIVE

THE OLD MAN
OF THE MOUNTAIN

"HI, MOMMA. This is Annie."

"He's gone," she says, sadly.

"Who's gone?"

"The old man," she replies.

"Daddy?" I ask.

"He's gone."

"To work?" I ask.

"No. He's gone. . . . [pause] . . . The old man."

Now I'm confused. I try again.

"I'll call back later when Daddy gets home," I say softly. "I love you, Momma."

"You're not supposed to call when he's sleeping," she says. "I can't get up."

"Okay, I'll call after your nap. I love you."

Later I hear the news. The Old Man of the Mountain fell in the night. Susie is right, once again. The Old Stone Face slid off in the night, a pile of granite crumpled at the base of the mountain. Everyone is amazed, filled with shock and awe. Life as we know it, carved in stone, has slipped away.

New Hampshire is The Granite State, solid as a rock. But now, the world we thought would never change is gone in the morning. Change is the only constant in our lives.

ॐ

My father adapts to the changes day by day, week by week. Slowly, he is coming to terms with the bedrock in his life shifting. My parents were married on April 30, 1948. They spent their first summer together working on Sel Hannah's farm in Franconia under the watchful eye of the Old Man of the Mountain.

The summer before, after he returned home from World War II to Dartmouth, my father was a hutman for the Appalachian Mountain Club at the Greenleaf Hut on Mount Lafayette. He was courting my mother, who was working with her twin sister, Sally, at the Hannah farm down in the village.

All summer long, Malcolm hauled the food for the AMC guests in a heavy pack on his back up the steep trail to the hut. After serving dinner, he would run down to town carrying a cake for his evening rendezvous with Susie. To this day, he still holds the record for the fastest ascent from Franconia Notch to the Greenleaf Hut on the Bridle Path.

My father spent the happiest days of his life in the White Mountains of New Hampshire, skiing and hiking in the mountains, swimming and canoeing in the lakes and streams. As captain of the Dartmouth Ski Team, he raced every trail from Moosilauke to Tecumseh, hiking to the top before ski lifts were invented and schussing to the bottom on wooden skis with bear-trap bindings.

In 1955, Malcolm was a founder of Wildcat Mountain Ski Area, located in Pinkham Notch with a spectacular view of Mount Washington. Three generations of our family and friends have shared the thrill of skiing and ski racing at Wildcat over the past half century.

In 1977, Susie was a founder of the New England Ski Museum, at the base of Cannon Mountain in Franconia Notch. She worked tirelessly with a group of old skiing friends and former ski racers, raising money, collecting artifacts, and cataloging generations of ski memorabilia.

Now everyone in the ski world can enjoy the history of our sport, from the earliest days of skiing in Norway to the adventures of the Tenth Mountain Division in World War II. Every young New Hampshire ski racer can share the Olympic glory of Penny Pitou winning her silver medal in Squaw Valley and of Bode Miller dazzling the crowd to win silver in Salt Lake City.

My mother won the Women's Eastern Ski Championship in 1948, only months before she married my father and moved to England. In 1970, Susie was the "fastest woman over forty" in the NASTAR National Championships in Aspen, Colorado. In 1993, in her last ski race at the Schneider Cup at Cranmore, she beat her twin sister only a year before Sally died of cancer.

My father was the ski representative to the U.S. Olympic Committee when I was growing up in the 1960's. He was involved in selecting the Winter Olympic sites and officiating at the ski events. With their friends Bud and Mary Little, of Helena, Montana, my parents attended the Winter Olympics at Squaw Valley in 1960 and Innsbruck in 1964, and the FIS World Ski Championships in Chamonix in 1962.

My sister Debbie ski raced for Harvard and I raced for Dartmouth in the 1970s. Now the torch is passed to the next generation. We cheer from the finish line as our children challenge the hill. Debbie married her Harvard ski coach, Peter Carter.

Their oldest daughter, Ashley, raced for Williams in three NCAA championships. Maile skied on the Dartmouth Ski Team and Laurel is a star at Burke Mountain Academy, with our son Zach. Our son Travis still skis for the Wildcat Mountain Ski Team, racing with the Macomber grandchildren every weekend all winter long.

๛

At long last, Malcolm is truly becoming the old man of the mountain. His knees are worn out from seventy years of hiking the rocky trails and skiing in the White Mountains. In the 1990s, my father had two knee replacements and my mother had two hip replacements. Now, after months and months of caring for Susie night and day, Malcolm is hobbling around with a cane, feeling the pain in his limbs and the sadness in his heart.

To further complicate the mental and emotional challenges of Alzheimer's disease, my mother's brain is slowly slipping away, resulting in a steady decline in her motor skills caused by "atrophy of the frontal lobe."

When I first discussed the news with my father, he was relieved, saying, "at least she didn't have a stroke." I did not have the heart to tell him that a stroke would have been one debilitating incident, whereas atrophy of the brain is a long, slow, steady decline.

In the beginning, the loss started in her right hand. Susie had difficulty writing a note. Eventually, she could barely sign her name. The last time we went shopping, I remember looking at the sales clerk, urging patience with my eyes, as my mother slowly, painstakingly signed her last signature.

As the months passed, the fingers on Susie's right hand began to curl up. She often sat with her hand in her lap, wrist bent, fingers curled, as though the hand that had changed ten thousand diapers, cooked for decades on end, and written a lifetime of speeches and songs was worn out and ready to rest.

Her physical disability spread from her right hand up her arm to her shoulder. Over time, we realized that she was losing muscle control in her right leg as well. Day by day, week by week, we learned to adjust as Susie lost the capacity to cope with the "activities of daily living."

My mother adapted with grace and courage. Right-handed her entire life, we barely noticed when Susie switched to eating with her left hand. But everything in her life now takes more time, more effort, more planning.

Susie's routine of brushing her teeth with one hand is a study in patience and perseverance. I remember on our camping trip out West in 1963, the summer I turned seven, when my mother taught us the trick of brushing our teeth with one cup of water.

Now I watch in awe as she swishes the brush in a cup of clean water and lays it on the counter. Then she picks up the tube and squeezes the toothpaste onto the brush. She sets down the tube, picks up the brush and slowly brushes her teeth with her left hand. Next she sets down the brush and picks up the cup of clean water to take a drink. She rinses her mouth and spits the water into the sink with a chuckle. Then she swishes the brush in the cup of clean water and pours the milky water down the sink.

Susie repeats the process to take her pills three times a day. First she fills a cup of clean water and sets it on the counter. Then she takes a pill in her left hand and pops it into her mouth. Next she lifts the cup and takes a drink. She swallows the pill and sets down the cup. Then she picks up the next pill and repeats the routine five or six times until all of the pills are gone.

Malcolm observes the changes in Susie's life with respect and admiration, encouraging her to do all that she can for herself, yet waiting patiently to help at any moment. Over time, my mother faces challenges dressing herself and coping in the bathroom. Peacefully, patiently, my father learns to remind her to start with the right sleeve first as he helps with her shirt or sweater or coat. They develop their own routine, one sleeve at a time.

"I've learned to start dressing a half hour before we go out," Malcolm reports, a habit I remember well with toddlers in snowsuits. The analogy comparing Alzheimer's disease to raising a child in reverse is uncannily accurate as my mother slips from dressing herself to being dressed, from coping in the bathroom to using Depends, from driving and walking on her own to sitting in a wheelchair, watching the world pass by.

Slowly, peacefully, patiently, my parents lead the way, teaching us to face the changes in their life. The bedrock is shifting once again. The Old Man of the Mountain slipped away in the night. The world as we knew it will never be the same. Change is the only constant in our lives.

CHAPTER TWENTY-SIX

'Day is Done'

WHERE WE LIVE, the world turns a different color for every season. Spring is filled with brilliant greens mixed with bright pink and yellow. The sky peeks through with a sparkling blue. It's beautiful, and sometimes overwhelming, like life, I suppose.

This is a story of a life filled with color, brilliant, bright, dazzling, and sometimes overwhelming. My parents have lived a beautiful life, like a party, with a long, slow dance at the end. Nobody wants the party to end. Every life is a story worth telling. This is our story, the story of our last dance.

Welcome to spring in New England, filled with color. One first big splash, as the leaves burst forth on the trees, the sun comes out, and the temperature finally rises after a long cold winter. In all its beauty, spring is a time to hold hope close to your heart. For every time there is a season. This is our season.

Now when someone on Main Street or in the State House asks "How's your mother?" I have the words to tell her story. "She's doing fine, but have you heard? She moved into a nursing home in February. She is in a wheelchair now. She can't speak, but she stays cheerful. My mother is safe and secure, surrounded by love. Thank you for asking."

༝

May 2004 arrives with a heat wave. The temperature soars, and by midday the daffodils are open to the sun. The boys finally wear shorts to school. The day is beautiful. After a long, bitter cold winter, the sight of bright red tulips, pink azaleas, and yellow forsythia brings hope back into our lives. Spring is a season of new beginnings. Spring holds promise close to our hearts.

A year ago, in the spring of 2003, Susie began to fall occasionally. As her right leg lost muscle strength, she lost her balance. We learned to hold her left arm firmly under the elbow and to support her getting up from a chair or into the car. At home, Susie held on tenaciously with her strong left hand to the railings that Donald had mounted on the walls. Malcolm walked along slowly, always at her side, ready with a helping hand.

Despite their challenges, my parents still enjoyed a busy life, with daily drives in the countryside and occasional evenings out for dinner or the theater. Then in late May 2003, as I escorted my mother through the crowd after a show at the Capitol Center for the Arts, she fell on the sidewalk next to the curb. As I turned to look over my shoulder to see Malcolm's car pull up to the curb, I felt Susie start to sway. In slow motion, she slipped from my grasp and crumpled in a heap at my feet.

Friends helped me get her back on her feet. Susie seemed fine, if not slightly embarrassed, as we helped her into the car. She smiled and waved as they drove off, but I realized that we were entering a new chapter in our lives. Our journey back in time was now in the toddler stage. Safety became an issue in Susie's world.

⤳

While our family loves winter and skiing in the mountains, my father lives for the spring and for summers on Newfound Lake. Malcolm comes alive with daylight savings time, counting the hours of sunshine in the day and dreaming of sunsets from the Pasquaney porch.

My father spends the winter making plans for Cousins Camp with hiking expeditions and family traditions at the lake. Then in May he takes down the shutters, sweeps off the porch and announces on Memorial Day that summer is officially here. Fun is waiting to happen.

The summer of 2003, Malcolm savored every moment at the lake, surrounded by family and friends, soaking in the sun and good times together. In late June, our family gathered for ten days of Cousins Camp, swimming across the lake, playing tennis and waterskiing, and hiking up Mount Washington for an overnight at the AMC Lakes of the Clouds hut.

Susie sat peacefully in a rocking chair on the porch, soaking up the love and attention flowing her way. Malcolm rocked slowly by her side, talking, laughing, sharing old stories and creating new memories, one sunset at a time.

One by one, we learned to help Susie get around and manage the challenges in her life. We took turns holding her by the elbow, slowly, step by step, navigating the stairs in the big house and the paths through the woods. Everyone learned to help her to the bathroom and in and out of bed.

My sisters and I developed a new intimacy with our mother, bathing her and washing her hair in the morning and tucking her into bed at night. Rather than dwell on what was lost in our lives, we focused on what was left in her life. As we kissed her on both cheeks and gazed into her sparkling eyes, passion, patience and perseverance soaked into our lives.

We celebrated the Fourth of July with dozens of McLane cousins, swimming and playing tennis, eating and singing songs, laughing and enjoying life. For fifty years, Susie entertained the crowds of cousins and guests graciously and efficiently. Now it takes a dozen of us to replace her in the kitchen, feeding the crowd and keeping the house humming with activity.

Susie pronounces the festive dinner "excellent," one of the few words left to her, superlative to the end. After the meal, we sing patriotic songs long into the night, mindful of the threat of war around the world, searching for peace in our hearts at home.

As we watch the brilliant red sun set over the shimmering blue water, glowing pink on the distant hills, we sing in unison with Susie at the center of our universe:

> *Day is done,*
> *gone the sun,*
> *from the hills,*
> *from the lake,*
> *from the sky.*
> *All is well,*
> *safely rest,*
> *God is nigh.*

Susie sings along, mouthing the words, smiling and feeling the love surround her. Our voices echo across the lake and into the granite hills beyond.

As night falls, the stars twinkle in the sky above. The moon rises from the mountain ridge across the lake. As darkness descends upon our world, fireworks burst forth from the heavens, falling through the night to the shimmering black lake, sparkling with the reflection of color and light.

THE LAST DANCE

Thy kingdom come.
Thy will be done.
On Earth
as it is in Heaven.

If there is a Heaven, let this be ours, surrounded by sunsets and songs. If this is our Heaven, let love surround us all, let there be peace in our hearts and in her soul. Let there be peace in our world. Amen.

CHAPTER TWENTY-SEVEN

'On Earth,
as it is in Heaven'

*A*s the summer of 2003 came to an end, my
parents' life became more and more difficult. My mother lost her
balance more often. She began to fall from time to time. We worried more and coped less, knowing in our hearts that their days
living together were coming to an end. How do you talk to your
parents about the end of a fifty-five-year marriage? How do you
arrange for a future without hope or promise? How do you plan
ahead when the end of an era is near?

Throughout my mother's illness, my father continued to
travel the world, taking respite trips every six months to recover
from the strain of care giving. Susie stayed at The Birches while
he was away. In April 2003, he took my son Travis on a
steamship trip down the Mississippi River. Then in October,
Malcolm and his brother Charles took the American Orient

Express train across the South, from Washington, D.C. to San Diego, then visited Donald in Seattle. Each time, Susie adjusted to her new world while Malcolm was away, but she was relieved to be home with him when he returned.

꒳ꙫ

The winter of 2004 was bitter cold in New Hampshire. My mother was finally in a wheelchair. Getting her out and about became more and more difficult. We managed to carry Susie into our house for the family Christmas celebration. Malcolm even took her overnight to the new AMC lodge in Crawford Notch.

Then in January, the temperature dropped below-zero for weeks at a time. My mother rarely left the house. My sisters and I visited whenever we could, bringing food and good cheer. But as their world closed in around them, the challenges of daily living took a toll on both my parents.

By February, my father was walking with a cane. He finally scheduled a hip replacement operation for the end of March. My son Travis broke his leg ski racing. The three of us were quite a sight grocery shopping Friday afternoons at Shaw's. Malcolm and Travis rode around in motorized shopping carts, while I directed traffic in the aisles.

Meanwhile, Susie could barely get out of bed, gripping the railing with her strong left hand and walking unsteadily, with Malcolm holding her up by the right elbow, step by step, day by day, slowly, cautiously, just getting by.

In late February 2004, Malcolm was planning to join friends from California on a respite trip to Mexico. As we arranged for Susie to return to The Birches while he was away, my father and I realized that she needed assistance now with all of the "activities of daily living." We knew that the program at The Birches was no longer suitable for her long-term needs.

As we talked about my mother's future, my father slowly came to the conclusion that he could not care for her at home when he returned from Mexico. He finally suggested that I look for a nursing home where Susie could stay, at least until he recovered from hip surgery.

While my father was in Mexico, I toured several nursing homes, searching for the people and program that would best serve my mother's physical and emotional needs. We were fortunate to find a bed, at least in the short term, at Havenwood, a private, non-profit nursing home in Concord.

In the end, we were blessed with good timing and good fortune. Debbie came to help move Susie for her week at The Birches. Then when my father came home from Mexico, Robin came to help move Susie to Havenwood, where she settled in peacefully to a comfortable routine with new faces and friends every day.

The week after his hip surgery in March, Malcolm even stayed in the bed next to Susie at Havenwood to recuperate and begin his rehabilitation. He was pleased and impressed by the competence and compassion of the staff. In time, my father began to understand the magnitude of my mother's disability. He realized the limits on his ability to care for her at home.

Day by day, family and friends came to visit Susie as she settled into her new life. Havenwood is affiliated with Heritage Heights retirement community, where many of my parents' friends from Concord have moved over the years. My mother is recognized by residents and staff on a daily basis. She loves the attention. Everyone loves her good cheer.

ॐ

My mother feels safe and secure in her new surroundings. Everyone is relieved. As we watch the staff care for her with grace and dignity, our uncertainty and fear about the future are slipping away. My father can let go of the burden of his responsibility as her primary caretaker. Now he can focus on his role as her husband, visiting every day, living in the moment, loving her one day at a time.

In May 2004, Susie settled into a permanent room on Memory Lane, the wing of the nursing home designed for dementia and Alzheimer's patients. The staff are well trained, tuning in to the individual needs of every resident, accommodating their lives one day at a time.

Malcolm visits every day, often in the afternoon when he can push Susie in her wheelchair down to the snack bar for an ice-cream cone. Robin and Debbie come by on the weekends. Alan came with daffodils from his garden on Mother's Day. I stop in a few times each week, before or after work, to take Susie for a walk in the garden.

Once when I visited early in the morning, Susie was still in bed, with two aides dressing her and getting her up for the day. I chatted with the women as they rubbed my mother's legs and feet with lotion, combed her hair, and put ointment on her lips and cream on her face.

"Momma," I said with a smile, "you ended up in a spa!"

Susie laughed with me. Then she smiled at her new friends. After fifty-five years devoted to caring for her husband and family, my mother is content to have these two kind and compassionate women caring for her. She deserves to rest. We are blessed.

‿ℑ‿

Today is our first walk outside in the sunshine. Susie spent most of the winter indoors, at home with my father in the coldest months, then here at the nursing home. Now spring is here again. The day is warm. The sun is bright.

The sun feels warm on our skin. The brilliant blue sky shines through the deep green leaves overhead. Pink tulips and yellow daffodils peak through the bright green grass below. Everywhere we look, our world is painted shades of green with splashes of bright colors.

"Look up, Momma, look at the clouds," I say, pointing up to the fluffy white clouds in the blue sky above.

My mother leans back in her wheelchair and smiles, with a look of surprise. Has she forgotten about clouds? I wonder. What goes on in her mind these days?

Our journey back in time with my mother continued through the winter and spring. Now Susie seems like a small child, marveling at the clouds and the beauty in her new world. I am blessed to share in her wonder.

"Momma, look at the robin," I say softly, watching her face turn toward the bird hopping across the grass. Then a gray squirrel scurries up a tree. Her head turns again. Her eyes slowly focus. My mother stares in amazement as the squirrel turns to watch her. She listens to a crow cackle from a branch above. Susie is attentive to her world, taking it all in, feeling nature surround her once again.

꒳

As the path winds around the corner of a row of independent-living apartments, we come upon a lovely white-haired woman planting pansies in her yard. We talk briefly about her recent trip to France. We admire the pansies planted in a border pattern along her walkway.

Suddenly, she looks down at my mother in the wheelchair, peering into her eyes, seeing her face for the first time since we began talking.

"You look just like Susan McLane!" she exclaims.

My mother begins to laugh, as I say, "This is . . . she is . . . Susan McLane."

The lovely woman leans down and takes my mother's hand in hers. She looks deep into her eyes, with a warm smile and an open heart.

"We are honored to have you living here at Havenwood," she says smiling, with reverence in her voice.

"You have done so much in the lives of women and families," she says, looking intently into my mother's face. "You have done so much for our whole community."

Still holding my mother's hand, she turns to look up at me.

"You have a remarkable family," she says with a smile.

My mother is beaming now, her head held high, her eyes sparkling, her face smiling. This woman's life is my mother's world. As I take in the scene, her life living in a retirement community, traveling to France, planting pansies, I see Susie's world in a whole different light.

Stopping by her home today, I wonder how this woman's world has changed over the years and who will ever tell her story. Then I realize that this story is for her, and for every woman or man whose life has been shaped by growing older, travelling the world, appreciating the beauty of nature, and by the everyday cares of making the world a better place for us all.

Behind my sunglasses, tears flow down my cheeks as I try to respond.

"You are so kind. Thank you." I say with a smile. "We will come see your pansies every week."

As we continue on our way down the path, my mother watches the world go by, knowing in her heart that she has made a difference in the lives of others, knowing that she has made the world a better place for all.

"You look just like Susan McLane!" I say, and she laughs. Then she tries to speak. I can barely make out the words. I lean down closer to her face.

"I can't speak, but I can listen," she says softly.

I kiss my mother on both cheeks. She is smiling now, with sparkling eyes full of pride and wonder. I am smiling, too, my eyes full of tears and love and laughter. I sing to her, quietly, peacefully:

> *Heaven,*
> *I'm in Heaven,*
> *and my heart beats so*
> *that I can hardly speak,*
> *and I seem to find*
> *the happiness I seek,*
> *when we're out together*
> *dancing cheek to cheek.*

Half of the grief about aging and Alzheimer's disease is learning to let go. We have learned to let go of the loss and to focus on the love and laughter. We have learned to be here with her, to be present in Susie's world.

Life is better to have loved and lost than never to have loved at all. We have learned to treasure our time together, our love for one another, our gift to each other.

> *Thy kingdom come.*
> *Thy will be done.*
> *On Earth*
> *as it is in Heaven.*

If there is a heaven, let this be hers, surrounded by sun and song. If this is her Heaven, let love surround her. Let there be peace in her heart and in her soul. Let there be peace in the world. Amen.

EPILOGUE

The girls take turns sitting with Susie on the porch, holding her hand, talking and laughing while she watches and listens. Her face glances up to the sky when she hears a bird chirping in the pine trees towering over the big house. She looks out on the water, peaceful and calm. Her eyes sparkle like the sun dancing on the dark shadows of the lake. Susie sits in silence, smiling on occasion, or staring out at her world, admiring the beauty of it all. One by one they sit, holding hands, telling stories, feeling her love surround them once again.

Malcolm sits in the rocking chair nearby, *The New York Times* folded in his lap. From time to time, he joins the conversation, but often he just watches his life unfold around him. Lunch is served out on the porch at the round green table under the yellow arches. The sun filters through the trees. A cool breeze stirs the air. Susie looks down at the lake, watching the girls paddling by in red canoes. She smiles and tries to wave, then looks back at us all, full of wonder once again.

Before she leaves in the wheelchair van with the nurse and driver, we sing songs on the porch in the afternoon sun. Susie tries to follow along as we sing old family favorites, *The Logger Lover, Clementine,* and *The Fox Went Out on a Chilly Night.* Then it is time to go. Everyone lines up for kisses on both cheeks. Susie is sleepy now and ready to rest. The music is winding down. The party is almost over.

৵

All week after her visit we share memories of Susie, laughing together about the good times gone by. We remember the sad times, too, as we each try to reconcile our feelings of love and loss. Each of us has our own perspective on her role in the family and her influence on our life.

Karissa, Maile, Carrie and Abi tell stories about marching for women and reproductive rights in Washington, D.C. this spring, inspired by their grandmother's lifelong devotion to the cause. Ashley appreciates Susie's optimism and good cheer, as she heads out into the world after graduating from Williams. Laura tells stories about living in Japan during college, while Marion calls from South Africa to report on observing the most recent elections.

Laurel and Zach share Susie's determination and competitive drive as they pursue their dreams in ski racing. Travis remembers his grandmother's generous spirit and delicious cooking. We all recall her nature scavenger hunts and birding expeditions to see the great blue heron and count the loons on the lake.

As our time together comes to an end, everyone laughs at Susie's favorite request of the grandchildren "to do one more chore" before leaving Pasquaney each summer—finish off the ice cream in the freezer.

Friends often ask about our visits with Susie and whether she recognizes us now. I am reminded of Lucia's response whenever I would ask about her mother: "She knows that I am someone who loves her very much." In our hearts, we all know that she is the one we love so much it hurts to let go.

We know that it will take the whole clan to carry on Susie's causes in the world, each one of us inspired by her courage and grace, her love and laughter. In her honor, we will make a difference in the world. One by one we will make the world a

better place for all. One by one we will finally find our way,
another day.

> Independence Day, July 4, 2004
> Newfound Lake, New Hampshire

'ANOTHER DAY'

James Taylor

Wake up Susie
put your shoes on
walk with me into this life
Oh, finally this morning
I'm feeling whole again
It was a hell of a night

Just to be with you
by my side
Just to have you near
in my sight
Just to walk awhile
in this light
Just to know that life goes on

Wake up Susie
put your shoes on
walk with me into this light

Another night has gone
Life goes on
Another dawn is breaking

Turn and face the sun
One by one
the world outside is waking

THE LAST DANCE

Morning light has driven away
all the shadows that hide your way
and night has given away to the promise of another day
Another day
another chance that we may finally find our way

Another day
The sun has begun to melt all our fears away
Another day
another day

Wake up Susie
put your shoes on
walk with me into this light

BOOK CLUB DISCUSSION FOR THE LAST DANCE

1. Based upon your own experience with aging and Alzheimer's disease (or any other illness), how did you relate to the various members of the McLane family in *The Last Dance*? Which character best describes your role? Do you recognize other members of your family? Explore themes of denial and candor that may have influenced your experience.

2. How was your experience similar? How was it different? Do you have a sense of why you react the way you do to the challenges you face? Does your reaction influence the experience of others?

3. Do you believe that Susan McLane's reaction to Alzheimer's may have influenced her experience with the disease? Explore the concept that "perception becomes reality" in your own life. Who controls your destiny? What literary characters come to mind?

4. How did communication in the McLane family change as Susie's Alzheimer's progressed? How has your family communication changed over time? Does your role in the family influence your pattern of communication and level of candor? Explore the concept of family secrets in your life.

5. *The Last Dance* explores the changing role of women over several generations. Which character relates best to your life story? What historical events have shaped the decisions in your life? Do you have regrets about decisions you have made in your life?

6. Susan McLane reacts to events in her life with the expression "and so, there it is." Do you consider her approach fatalistic or a realistic coping mechanism for facing adversity? How do you cope with adversity in your life?

7. What is your reaction to the expression "*One foot in the future, one foot in the past, and you are pissing on the present*"? How do events in your past, or plans for your future, impact upon the way you live your life every day?

8. Susan grew up an identical twin in a small community with a well-known father. How did these elements of her childhood influence her adult life? Explore the balance between private and public lives. How do these themes impact your life? What historic or literary characters come to mind?

9. *The Last Dance* could best be described as "herstory." How does this approach differ from classical forms of "history"? Which do you prefer? Why?

10. How did the natural world influence *The Last Dance*? Explore the impact of the changing seasons, the geography of New Hampshire, and the natural beauty of the land in the book. How does nature influence your life?

11. The events of September 11, 2001, profoundly influenced our lives. How have historical events changed your perspective on life? Explore the reaction of various characters in the book to changes in the world of politics and historical events. How have these same events (World War II, the Vietnam Era, September 11) changed your life or those in your family?

12. Susan and Malcolm McLane lived in England when they were first married and traveled the world throughout their lives. Explore the juxtaposition of creating a world view while living their entire lives in a small state surrounded by people they have known since childhood.

13. *"Change is the only constant in our lives."* Do you embrace change or do you prefer life to stay the same? How did the characters in *The Last Dance* react to the changes in their lives? Explore the metaphors for change (the Old Man of the Mountain, raising children and aging parents, the seasons) in the book.

14. Susan McLane has led "a meaningful life." She is "willing to die tomorrow." Explore your assessment of your own life and how that influences your approach to death and dying. Now explore how your approach to the end of life influences the way you lead your life every day.

15. Would you recommend *The Last Dance* to a friend or to someone in your family? Why? Would you tell them why before they read the book? How might their reaction differ from yours?

THE AUTHOR

Ann McLane Kuster grew up in Concord, New Hampshire, the youngest daughter in a prominent political family. After graduating from Dartmouth College in 1978, she worked on Capitol Hill for Congressman Pete McCloskey, traveling to the Middle East and southern Africa on congressional fact-finding missions. In 1984, Ann received her law degree from Georgetown University and returned to New Hampshire to practice in the McLane Law Firm in Manchester.

Ann is now a partner in the Concord law firm of Rath, Young and Pignatelli, P.A., where she has practiced since 1987, representing primarily health care and higher education clients in the New Hampshire Legislature. She maintains a private adoption practice and is a member of the American Academy of Adoption Attorneys.

Active in community service, Ann has raised funds for and served on the Boards of the United Way of Merrimack County, Child and Family Services of New Hampshire, the Tucker Foundation at Dartmouth College, the Capitol Center for the Arts, and The Women's Fund of New Hampshire. She currently serves on the Boards of the New Hampshire Charitable Foundation and Womankind Counseling Center. Ann is a member of the New Hampshire delegation to the 2004 Democratic National Convention in Boston.

Ann lives in Hopkinton, New Hampshire, with her husband Brad, who is a lawyer for the Conservation Law Foundation, and their two sons, Zach and Travis.